Total
Well Being

To: Susan
Best wishes on your
journey to Total Well Being
Jack E Young
1996

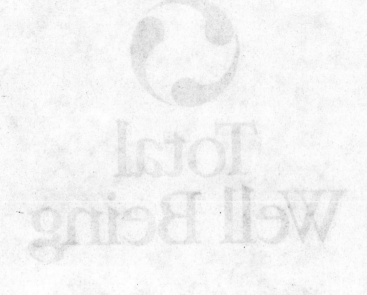

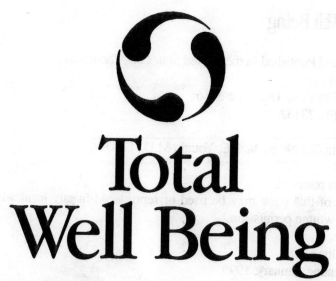

Total Well Being

Integrated Balance of Body, Mind and Spirit

By
Jack E. Young, M.D., Ph.D.
F.A.C.S.M., D.A.B.E.M.

Edited by Celia Straus

Total Well Being

Printed and Published in the United States of America by:
Tri Health, Inc.
1717 N Bayshore Dr., Suite 3936
Miami, FL, 33132

First Edition
First Printing, January, 1995

ISBN 0-9644716-0-4

Additional copies of Total Well Being may be obtained from:

Tri Health, Inc.
1717 N Bayshore Dr.
Suite 3936
Miami, Fl 33132

1-800 DR YOUNG (379 6864)

Dedication

I dedicate this work to the two most important people in my life
my daughter, Juli Gerlach and my son, Nathan Young.

Acknowledgments

I am extremely grateful to Celia Straus, the Editor of this book, who has been a constant source of encouragement, and who has molded my scientific jargon into user-friendly easy reading.

I would still be rewriting manuscripts of this book if it were not for Paula Black and Associates, Jane McGeary, Fran Wilson, Layne Mitchell and Lidia Leonard. Their belief in the principals of this work, their dynamic enthusiasm and talent made this book happen.

I am especially grateful to Nan Peacock who guided me through the writing of this book giving me both personal and professional support, and to the following people who read preliminary manuscripts of this book and offered critical and helpful feedback: Brian Clement, Dennis Devane, Martha Elmdorf, Carl Foster, Ph.D., Ted Feldman, M.D., Rose Harris, Eugene Lorenz, Laszlo Makk, M.D., Edward Reid, M.D., George Vegera, M.D., Gerard von Dohlen, and Jim and Joanne Young.

Although I am fully responsible for the content of the book, it would not be nearly so comprehensive, accurate or illustrative without the help of Tracy Herzog, Nathan Young, Rick Cabrera, and Jean Baton for their help in creating the exercise photography; Luis Feldman and Fine Arts for shooting the exercise photography; Ron Corso for his artistic photography which provided the cover; and Teri Vara for the medical illustrations.

In addition, I would like to extend my heartfelt thanks to HealthSouth Corporation, the staff at the Health and Fitness Institute at HealthSouth Doctors' Hospital, and, most important of all, the participants and patients who over the years have allowed me the opportunity to learn from them so that I could provide resources for other people to help themselves achieve Total Well Being.

Note To The Reader

The art and practice of medicine requires a one on one patient physician relationship. This book offers sound advice on how you can improve your physical fitness, nutrition and mental and spiritual well being. Unfortunately, since I do not have a physician patient relationship with you, I cannot assume the responsibility for your diagnosis or treatment. Therefore, at the slightest question or provocation of discomfort or injury I advise you to see your physician.

Table of Contents

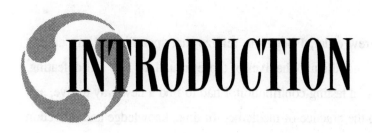

INTRODUCTION

Why Write This Book?

"Wow, Do I Feel Great!" I wouldn't have said that ten years ago . . . indeed, I could not have said that ten years ago . . . because, for most of my adult life, I followed the typical American lifestyle. I was obsessive and compulsive . . . a perfectionist . . . a workaholic with lousy nutrition . . . and virtually no physical activity. During my invincible twenties, I got by with this lifestyle. During my thirties, I would occasionally wake up feeling achy and tired and start thinking that maybe I was mortal after all. Then, I hit what I call the decay decade . . . my forties. I gradually began to get chronic indigestion, headaches, muscle and joint pains, unusual fatigue and a slew of other symptoms associated with my body's slow deterioration toward the degenerative diseases. Is this beginning to sound familiar? Well, I'd had enough; that's when I turned my life around.

Indeed, I am convinced that my life was planned to culminate in who I am today . . . that fate put together the events in my life to evolve one after another in order to bring me to the point of writing this book. As a boy, I nursed an invalid mother. After high school, I worked my way through undergraduate and graduate schools and became a University professor with awards for teaching. I was invited into a special medical school program from which I graduated in eighteen months . . . and afterwards worked for years in hospital emergency departments treating the sickest of people. In the past decade, I moved into preventive and sports medicine to treat patients at the opposite, healthy end of the medical spectrum.

NOTE:
Then, I hit what I call the decay decade . . . my forties.

As I grew older, I began to realize that spending all my energy trying to control my life and the lives of those around me was self-defeating. In order to make a lasting contribution, I had to find a new way to live, and then apply it to the practice of medicine. In time, knowledge and reflection gave me the wisdom to embrace the concept of total well being. I realized that my responsibilities as a physician . . . a healer . . . went way beyond a practice or group of patients. What I know now is that my life's experiences are gifts . . . gifts to share with you.

And this is why I wrote this book . . . to spark a flame in your life . . . like the one in mine . . . towards the freedom of being in control of your life in a new way. And, for those of you who are ready and willing, to guide you along the path I have taken to Total Well Being.

Why Should You Read This Book?

NOTE:
. . . I can give you the resources to help you change your life . . .

You may realize that you don't feel great, but chalk it up to age, stress, bad nutrition or not enough sleep. Do you want to change but aren't sure how to begin? Have you tried to change through countless diets and exercise programs but have never been able to keep it up? Change is hard! It takes a strong belief in yourself, knowledge of how to do it, role models, practice and, above all, <u>commitment</u>. I know that you can feel great, and that I can give you the resources to help you change your life . . . once and for all.

I assume that you desire change, but you need the motivating information to help you make that commitment and, most important of all, maintain it beyond the initial euphoria of trying something new. You may even be able to visualize what change you want to bring about . . . whether it's a slimmer, more muscular body . . . a more relaxed, happier demeanor . . . fewer aches and pains . . . more energy. This book provides you with a way to start changing with trust instead of fear. It gives you the concepts that form the basis for improving your physical, mental and spiritual well being.

How This Book Works

It is a scientific fact that our health is a continuum from wellness to disease. This book tells you how you can interrupt that slow progressive march, indeed preserve your health and prevent disease, by making certain lifestyle changes. Chapter 1, "America's Health Continuum," specifically describes the changes you can make to intervene in this march toward early illness and death. It explains why it's important to direct your energies toward a state of integrated balance between body, mind and spirit; which is the definition of total well being.

As you read, you will begin to understand the concepts of each of these areas of total well being and how to incorporate changes in your life to increase and improve each area. Chapter 1 ends with the premise that in our society the most practical approach to total well being is through your body.

Therefore, in Chapter 2, "Physical Fitness," I will discuss all the components of physical fitness, how exercise can improve your life, and show how you can use objective, no nonsense principles to improve your "physicalness." What you read here will generate an excitement and determination to exercise . . . to pay attention to your body by choosing

NOTE:
. . . our health is a continuum from wellness to disease.

activities that fit you and you alone. At the end of the chapter, I'll give you step by step instructions on when to obtain medical clearance for exercise, and then show you how to stretch, strengthen and do aerobic exercises properly and safely. This will get you started on your path to total well being.

However, physical fitness does not exist in a vacuum. Proper nutrition is also essential. Therefore, the focus of Chapter 3 is on nutrition. These days, nutritional advice is everywhere . . . most often in the guise of diet books. However, diet and nutrition are not the same thing. Proper nutrition combines science, simplicity, moderation and common sense. To make it easier for you, I show you how we should eat by creating a "Nutrition Continuum." This diagram demonstrates the fallacies of diet after diet . . . many of which I am willing to bet you've tried. Besides teaching you the basic concepts of good nutrition, I provide all the resources you need to combine proper nutrition with fitness.

Once you understand the body (physical fitness and nutrition), you are ready to begin the movement into the mind and spirit. The book ends with Chapter 4, "Mental and Spiritual Fitness." It is here that you will learn why and how you can change your belief system. I focus on the belief system because this deep-seated collection of experiences determines our attitudes, thoughts and personalities . . . all of which dictate our behaviors. In this chapter, I will give you a model of behavior modification that takes you from a projected vision of what you would like to change about yourself to its realization. This model gives you ways to realize your goals by first understanding what your goals really are, then substantiating them with models, reinforcing them with introspection and, finally, solidifying them with reflection. Again, I will give you clear, concise steps to achieve mental and spiritual wellness.

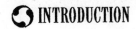

Why This Book Is User Friendly

Most wellness books on diet, exercise, stress management or spiritual enlightenment are written to be read, not used. This book is different. I have designed it so that you can refer to its pages again and again, using it more like a manual than a treatise on well being. For instance, as a teacher, I know that a picture is worth a thousand words. Therefore, I've included tables, figures, illustrations and photographs to display facts, data, concepts and exercises. There are tables to fill out and simple formulas to complete. At the end of Chapters 2, 3 and 4, you will get hands-on practical applications so you can start your journey now! Throughout the book, I've given you names of individuals, organizations and book titles to help you build your own self-help library. These resources are identified with a number in parentheses, (1), and are discussed at the end of each chapter. In addition, I've cited the most authoritative, up-to-date references regarding controversial topics or those I think you may want to pursue. References are indicated with a superscript, [1].

However, I want to caution you, that the scientific literature and statistics can be manipulated to prove any bias. This was clearly illustrated during the 1994 congressional hearings by the Health Committee on the use of tobacco in this country. The presidents of seven major tobacco producing companies used "scientific data" to (1) prove that the use of tobacco is not addicting, and (2) state unequivocally that there is no proof tobacco products cause cancer. Indeed, when you analyze the statistics used to perpetuate these outrageous lies, the numbers they utilize are perfectly legitimate. Therefore, if you want to verify the literature, use the references provided and their bibliographies to further search out the facts and decide for yourself.

> **NOTE:**
> *You can refer to these pages again and again, using it more like a manual than a treatise on well being.*

Your Path

NOTE:

*. . . an integrated
balance of
Body, Mind
and Spirit . . .
Total Well
Being . . .*

As I review the events in my life, it is clear that they have led me to writing this book for you. As a physician and teacher, I intend to provide you with the concepts to properly and safely improve your physical fitness and in so doing, help you move into mental and spiritual fitness. You will then arrive at an integrated balance of Body, Mind and Spirit . . . Total Well Being . . . so that you to can say each day of your life, "Wow, Do I Feel Great!"

1 AMERICA'S HEALTH CONTINUUM

Introduction

In looking back on the 1980's, it seems that many of us believed in the Billy Crystal, Saturday Night Live line, "It is better to look good than to feel good." We spent an inordinate amount of time, effort and money on our appearance, often at the detriment to our health. After a decade of starvation from crazy diets, injury from inaccurate and intense exercise, shrinking wallets from expensive club memberships, and dwindling storage space in our homes from the purchase of the latest thighmaster machine, Americans are still, for the most part, unfit.

Moreover, there's not a single one of us who is getting any younger, and the baby boomers are marching steadfastly into their fifties. Additionally, we are paying the price of soaring health care costs associated with our present health care system. Today, more than ever, it's critical that we take responsibility, not only for the way we look, but also for the way we feel.

If Ponce de Leon were alive today and searching for the fountain of youth, surely he would find it in the simple, safe approach to life . . . exercise, nutrition and contentment. Fulfillment in these areas will lead us all to a more productive, energetic life. What you will experience from a modicum of fitness is increased energy and a feeling of well being that will flow into every facet of your life, giving you the discipline necessary to achieve whatever it is you wish. If there were such a thing as a "miracle drug" it would be fitness and good health. This book will show you how to reach that end and we'll start with looking at what I call the Health Continuum, Figure 1.1.

The Health Continuum

NOTE:

. . .*we can make a difference by the way we live* . . .
our lifestyles.

A good way to understand your health relative to your life is to position yourself along this continuum.

Figure 1.1
THE HEALTH CONTINUUM

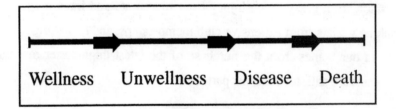

Wellness   Unwellness   Disease   Death

During our lives, our health begins with wellness . . . progresses to unwellness . . . then disease . . . and finally death. This is everyone's progressive process to their inevitable end. But, the quality of life is equally as important as the quantity of life, or pace of the progression. And, even though the stages along the way are variable for each of us as a result of our genetic predispositions, we can make a difference by the way we live . . . our lifestyles.

If we're willing to take control of our own lives, and our bodies, each of us can intervene and slow this progression down. The question is, how? How do we slow down this march that takes away the quality of our lives? In other words, how do we start to practice preventive medicine in our own lives?

The answers to these questions provide the underlying concepts of total well being which guide this book. Let's start by looking at our Health Continuum within the context of how doctors approached medicine and health in the past. For doctors and patients alike, comprehending where we've been, helps us to understand where we're going.

Disease Not Patients

Throughout most of this century, disease has been the focus of health care. Like Hippocrates, physicians have taken an allopathic approach to their profession, meaning that the treatment of disease involves therapies such as drugs, radiation and surgery. This approach became formalized in 1910 when, based upon the Flexner Report, the American Medical Association charged that doctors should follow a scientific approach in the training and practice of medicine (1). Indeed, physicians are incredibly conscientious, dedicated and hard working. It takes eleven years or more of intense study and devotion to the science of medicine just to get ready to practice. Physicians care about their patients twenty four hours a day seven days a week. I know, I've been in the trenches of emergency departments nights, weekends and holidays. However, the focus of our training deals with solving the symptoms of the problem rather than dealing with causes or the prevention of the problem. Disease, not people, is basically what we physicians have chosen to spend our lives studying, researching and treating.

NOTE:
Throughout most of this century disease has been the focus of health care.

The "Ole Gommer"

As a new intern, I will never forget one early morning making rounds on the wards of our county hospital. My team was waiting impatiently at the elevator when the door opened and we met a second team. Their resident, with an air of superiority, urged us to head over to West Wing 201 and examine the newly admitted "fascinoma." "It's a once-in-a-lifetime opportunity," he said. "And while you're there, make sure you check out his incredible X-rays. But hurry," he added, "the ole gommer's about to croak."

As our team hustled along, I couldn't help but voice my shock at the resident's unfeeling description of a dying man. What about the person himself . . . his family? When my concern was met with blank stares, I fell silent, confused and embarrassed at not fitting in with the doctors whom I revered. I began to wonder if this was what being a physician was all about?

As time went on, like most of my colleagues, I developed a policy against becoming too close to my patients. We embraced it as "self preservation" because getting to know patients as people hurt too much if we weren't successful in treating their diseases.

Of course, in those days working in a busy county hospital, I had little choice but to focus on the immediate pathology of my patients. The number of people we had to treat, and the severity of their conditions left little time for anything else. In addition, I paid little attention to the financial side of medicine. That's how we were trained in those days.

The "Golden Age" of Medicine

For decades physicians were mandated to provide whatever was needed, for whomever needed it and whenever it was needed. This was, in large part, due to Medicare and Medicaid which was instituted in the sixties. The result of these government entitlement programs was a healthcare system bogged down by inefficiency and skyrocketing costs (2-4).

In the past decade, however, the established medical communities have gradually shifted away from myopic disease-oriented treatments toward patient-driven holistic practices. One example is the National Institutes of Health's Office of Alternative Medicine which funds research on the impact of healing by alternative practices such as the mind/body connection, meditation, acupuncture and nutritional therapy. There are now many renowned and well respected physicians who practice alternative forms of medical therapy (5-7).

For me, the change occurred when I became interested in the study and practice of preventive and sports medicine. As a twenty year veteran of the emergency department, I treated thousands of cardiac and musculoskeletal conditions. Gradually, I became convinced there had to be a better approach to health care than just the treatment of disease.

However, the orthodox medical definition of preventive medicine falls far short of the true meaning of the words. To explain this concept, let's look at Figure 1.2, The ED Health Continuum. Allopathic medicine intervenes on the continuum at a point I call "ED," or Early Detection.

NOTE:
For decades physicians were mandated to provide whatever was needed, for whomever needed it and whenever it was needed.

Figure 1.2
THE ED HEALTH CONTINUUM

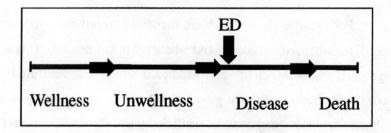

Is early detection truly prevention? What about all those people who fall into the unwell category and have vague, ubiquitous symptoms with diagnoses such as headache, fatigue, arthritis, indigestion, hypoglycemia, candidiasis and on and on? Orthodox medicine labels people in this category as having "psychosomatic symptoms," "supratentorial reactions" or, just simply, exhibiting crazy behavior. Yet, these people are not well! What are we missing?

After further years of study and experience, I became convinced that a more holistic approach to medicine would serve a greater number of people. Thus, it was with considerable anticipation and excitement that nine years ago I, along with other pioneers in our hospital, created the now famous Health and Fitness Institute of HealthSouth Doctors' Hospital in Coral Gables, Florida.

As Medical Director of the Institute, I supervise programs in exercise, nutrition and stress management. These programs are designed to help people modify their lifestyles leading toward wellness. I provide medical care for a variety of community sporting events and function as a team physician for the University of Miami Hurricanes and the professional arena football team, the Miami Hooters. This gives me even more opportunities to practice preventive and sports medicine, helping not just athletes, but hundreds of people find better lives through health and fitness.

I still believe in orthodox medicine . . . even super medical specialization and hi-tech medicine. Indeed, modern medicine plays a unique role by rendering health care that no other form of treatment can provide. To those who blame orthodox medicine for our health care crisis, (see 3), I say, "NO! Let's not throw the baby out with the bath water!" The term holistic means to utilize all helpful means of health care to treat patients and to place more emphasis on the preventive approach to health care.

So, the practice of true Preventive Medicine is intervention at a point "PM" on the Health Continuum, Figure 1.3. Preventive medicine intervenes before people become unwell.

NOTE:
Preventive medicine intervenes before people become unwell.

Figure 1.3
THE PM HEALTH CONTINUUM

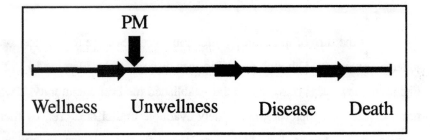

America's Killers

But, how do we intervene? What practical steps do we take? The answer lies in a simple graph, yet one that is packed with insightful information, Figure 1.4.

Figure 1.4
THE LEADING CAUSES OF DEATH
in America During the 1900's*

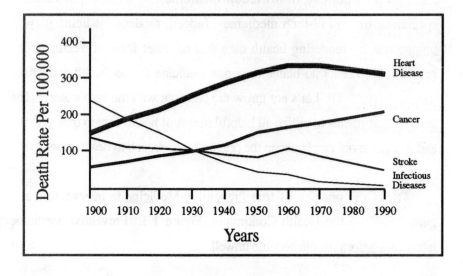

*Adapted from: Stallones, R.A. Scientific American. *The Rise and Fall of Ischemic Heart Disease.* 1980; 243:53-59.

At the turn of the century, infectious diseases were the number one killer in America. Although penicillin was discovered by Fleming in 1928, like many new ideas presented to the established medical community, it was not accepted and, therefore, not widely available until 1943. Yet, by then, despite such a momentous discovery, the infectious disease curve had dropped by more than three quarters. What accounted for the decreased death rate from infectious diseases? Simple, common sense practices such as people washing their hands and household items, avoiding direct contact with infectious patients and improvements in public health and sanitation. In short, people taking care of themselves before disease strikes!

This is what preventive medicine is all about! And, doesn't it make sense that greater emphasis on prevention would continue to work for us today? The answer, of course, is yes! Our society saw the total number of deaths from infectious diseases drop drastically by practicing rudimentary preventive medicine. It only makes sense that we would see a far greater reduction in death from all diseases by taking a <u>proactive</u> approach by adopting healthy lifestyles. And, as you will see, preventive medicine such as the lifestyle changes associated with exercise and diet can reduce the diseases that kill fifty percent of Americans. In other words, it is within <u>your power</u> to avoid the leading causes of death! For example, thousands of cancer cases are related to life-style practices; 35% with diet and 30% with tobacco use.[1]

Enemy Number One

Look again at Figure 1.5 and this time identify the leading causes of death today . . . Heart Disease, Cancer and Stroke. There are incredible lessons hidden in these three curves. For instance, ask yourself, "What kind of cancer causes the greatest number of deaths?" Remember, these graphs report both sexes and all ages of Americans.

You might respond with colon or breast cancer, but, the facts are that it is lung cancer. And, get this, 80-85% of deaths from lung cancer are directly attributable to smoking.[2] Is that simply a random association? Colon cancer, the second leading cause of cancer death, has been unequivocally linked to a high fat, low fiber diet.[3] Breast cancer may also be related to diet.[4,5]

Can you imagine what impact intervention at the point "PM" on our Health Continuum could have on these cancers? Preventive medicine could reduce the suffering of millions of Americans and reduce the medical costs in this country by billions . . . every year!

NOTE:
. . . the leading causes of death today . . . Heart Disease, Cancer and Stroke.

Killers Number One and Three: Atherosclerosis

Now, let's consider the cause of the first and third killers today . . . Heart Disease and Stroke. When doctors refer to heart disease, they could mean any number of problems associated with the heart, including valve abnormalities, rhythm disturbances, muscle weaknesses or vessel disease. But, the heart condition that kills most of us is plaque build-up in the arteries that feed our hearts. The scientific name for plaque build-up is atherosclerosis, which is what most people refer to as heart disease.

Minimal plaque itself is only a prelude to future disaster, but moderate plaque can diminish the flow of nutrients and oxygen to our cells leading to what is called "ischemia," see Figure 1.5. Ischemia can cause memory loss, poor vision, muscle aches and pains, digestive abnormalities and other problems, depending upon the organs involved. If ischemia occurs in the heart, it causes the heart muscle to go into spasms which is called angina pectoris, or "angina" for short. Decreased blood flow to the brain may cause a temporary dysfunction of the central nervous system called a transient ischemic attack, or TIA.

When our blood vessels become totally blocked, the cells fed by those vessels die, which is called "infarction," Figure 1.5. Since the scientific name for the heart is myocardium, when heart muscles die it is diagnosed as a myocardial infarction ("MI"). If brain cells die because of a lack of blood flow, it is a stroke.

Figure 1.5
THE PATHOPHYSIOLOGY OF ATHEROSCLEROSIS

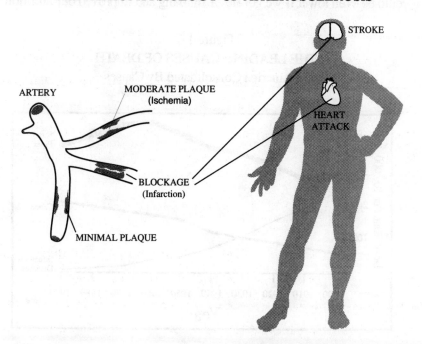

To summarize, atherosclerosis is plaque build-up in our arteries which blocks the flow of nutrients to our cells. This may lead to ischemia which produces mild to moderate symptoms such as angina . . . or, with further obstruction, it may lead to infarction or cell death. The greater the area or number of cells that die, especially in vital organs such as our hearts or brains, the greater the chance that we will die.

"Rusty Pipes"

Now, let's look at the modern causes of death in more detail, Figure 1.6. This graph <u>combines</u> the curves for heart disease and stroke since they have a common cause . . . atherosclerosis. The curve, then, represents what I call "Rusty Pipes," and it practically soars off the chart!

NOTE:
. . . heart disease and stroke . . . have a common cause . . . atherosclerosis.

The next cause of death, cancer, drops way down on the graph, and it could be even lower if we got rid of smoking and improved our nutrition.

Figure 1.6
THE LEADING CAUSES OF DEATH
in America Consolidated By Causes

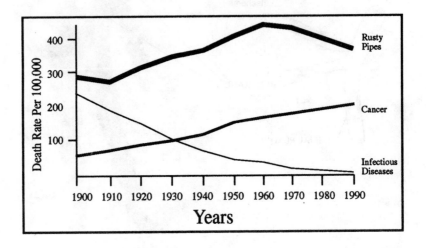

Here is what we've learned so far:

1. Plaque build-up in our arteries presently accounts for the majority of deaths (quantity) and explains to a large extent the cause of unwell symptoms (quality) in the lives of Americans.

2. Prevention, or changing our lifestyles, plays the most important role in keeping us well, thereby decreasing the incidence of diseases that disable or kill us.

NOTE:
. . . prevention can prolong and improve your life.

Intervening at point PM on your Health Continuum through prevention can prolong and improve your life. However, before you can intervene, you need to know what risks are associated with these leading causes of death so that you can be very specific about what you want to change. Do it now! The changes you make in your behavior will enable you to achieve the best quality and quantity of life . . . total well being.

Risk Factors

Follow Table 1.1 as I discuss the risk factors associated with that number one killer, Rusty Pipes. I listed them in order of importance based upon my clinical experience. That is, those at the top of the list are more likely to predict your chances of developing a heart attack or stroke.

Table 1.1
RISK FACTORS FOR ATHEROSCLEROSIS

Description	Definition	Normal*
MAJOR		
1. Family History	Parent or Sibling under age 55	N/A
2. Cigarette Smoking	The greater the number smoked/day and the longer the years smoked, the greater the risk	None
3. Total Blood Cholesterol	240 (mg/dl)	<150 No Risk 150-200 Mild Risk 201-239 Mod. Risk > 240 High Risk
4. High Blood Pressure (mmHg)	160/90 on at least 2 different occasions	Diastolic < 90 Normal 90-104 Mild 105-114 Mod. >115 Severe
5. Diabetes Mellitus	Insulin Dependent	N/A
6. Physical Inactivity	Risk decreases by 1/2 with 2,500 Cal/week	N/A
MINOR		
7. Obesity	20% over ideal Body Weight	N/A
8. Psychological Stress	Hostile Type A	N/A
9. Age	N/A	N/A

* < = less than, > = greater than

The Major Risks

The first six risks are what we call major risk factors. That means each one, as defined, stands alone in its statistical relationship to atherosclerosis, while the minor risk factors need to be paired together in order to be statistically significant.

Risk 1: Family History

NOTE:

By exploring your genetic heritage. . . you can learn a tremendous amount about your own potential for illness.

Let's start with the most significant risk, Family History. Check yourself on this one! To be positive for this risk, either your parents or siblings must have been diagnosed with atherosclerosis before age 55. They could have been diagnosed as having had a heart attack, stroke or claudication, which is a condition where the plaque builds up in the arteries of their legs so that they have severe pain with physical activity.

Your family history is the best predictor as to what diseases you may develop, as well as the rate of progression along your Health Continuum. The best action you can take to decrease your vulnerability to inherited diseases is to investigate your family history. By exploring your genetic heritage, particularly the maternal or paternal side of the family you most resemble, you can learn a tremendous amount about your own potential for illness. This does not require genetic testing of any kind. Your own personal research will give you indications of what lifestyle changes you should make in order to avoid those diseases that are handed down from generation to generation in your family.

Risk 2: Cigarette Smoking

The second major risk factor, the most important one over which you have total control, is smoking cigarettes. There is no definitive cut-off for when this becomes a major risk since the effects of nicotine and tars are slow and progressive. The greater the number of cigarettes smoked each day over the longer number of years, the greater the risk.

NOTE:
Nicotine addiction has been equated to the worst of drug addictions.

This addiction raises havoc with your arteries because it contributes to plaque formation which interferes with oxygen transport in your blood. In addition, nicotine is a potent vasoconstrictor, meaning that it causes your blood vessels to constrict, thereby further reducing the blood flow and the delivery of nutrients to your cells. Thus, smokers continually put themselves in double jeopardy for having a heart attack or stroke.

For instance, imagine eating a big meal topped off with dessert and coffee . . . sugar and caffeine combine to cause your heart to beat faster. Then, consider what happens when you smoke and add nicotine to this scenario. Remember, nicotine has already contributed to the obstruction of the flow of blood by increasing plaque formation. Now, it acutely constricts the arteries feeding your heart just when your heart muscle is beating faster and under greater demand for nutrients and oxygen. The result of this combination is often fatal. Needless to say, the best way to change this risk factor is <u>simple</u> . . . STOP SMOKING!

I said simple, <u>not easy</u>. Nicotine addiction has been equated to the worst of drug addictions. There are many successful smoking cessation programs such as group sessions, hypnosis, acupuncture and the nicotine patch. These programs often motivate people to make the psychological switch necessary to take action and be responsible for themselves. Indeed, one of the best, long-lasting approaches is to stop "cold turkey." In fact, <u>self</u> <u>cure</u> from smoking and other addictive behaviors appears to be more effective long-term than therapeutic treatment alone.[6] Those who are successful finally decide, for whatever reason, to just quit! This decision-making power that we possess offers a profound lesson for our total well being.

No matter what our external stimuli, successful behavioral changes must come from within us.

Risk 3: Total Blood Cholesterol

NOTE:

Total cholesterol levels greater than 240 mg/dl are seriously high . . .

The third risk is an elevated blood cholesterol level. Keep in mind that cholesterol itself is not harmful. In fact, it is essential as a precursor to the synthesis of steroid hormones such as cortisone, estrogen and testosterone. Cholesterol is also incorporated into connective tissue which forms the building blocks that help hold our cells and organs together. However, too much cholesterol in the blood leads to the build-up of plaque that causes rusty pipes.

Total cholesterol levels greater than 240 mg/dl are seriously high, while levels below 150 mg/dl are associated with no risk. Yet, these lower levels provide enough of this essential substance to promote healthy tissue.

There are two kinds of cholesterol . . . the good (HDL) cholesterol and the bad (LDL) cholesterol. When I discuss blood cholesterols with my patients, I tell them to remember that the good kind is HDL . . . High Density Lipoprotein . . . High, Heaven, Good. One of my patients said, "Oh, the H stands for Happy, Healthy." The LDL . . . Low Density Lipoprotein . . . stands for Low Down Lousy.

If your total cholesterol is less than 200 mg/dl, that's OK, even though you would be at lower risk if it was below 150 mg/dl. But, if your cholesterol is greater than 200 mg/dl, you should ask your doctor for a lipid profile to get a breakdown of the two types in your blood.

Your Lipid Profile

It is important to know your lipid profile because the LDL fraction plays a role in the initiation of plaque formation along the inner layer of our arteries. Optimal LDL cholesterol levels are below 130 mg/dl, while dangerously high levels are in excess of 160 mg/dl. The protective HDL fraction is like a biochemical pac man; it gobbles up extra LDL cholesterol. HDL cholesterol levels above 50 mg/dl are considered favorable, but it really depends on the level of HDL cholesterol in relation to the total cholesterol . . . the Ratio.

The Cholesterol Ratio

The ratio is calculated by dividing the total cholesterol by the HDL cholesterol. Now, get ready, I'm going to ask you a math question. Notice, that total cholesterol is a larger number than its component, HDL. Therefore, we come up with a whole number, for example $200 \div 50 = 4$. Also, notice that the total cholesterol is in the numerator and the HDL is in the denominator. Here's your math question; do we want a higher or lower number in the ratio? Give up? The answer is, lower.

Putting it All Together

If you need to have your lipid profile determined, compare it with the following standards, Figure 1.7.

Figure 1.7
STANDARDS FOR LIPID PROFILE

Measurement	Range (mg/dl)		
	Ideal	Moderate Risk	High Risk
Total Cholesterol	<	200 – 240	>
LDL Cholesterol	<	130 – 160	>
Ratio	<	3.5 – 6.0	>
Analysis	Great	Lifestyle Change	See Your Doctor

If your numbers are in the Ideal range, great! If they are in the Moderate Risk range, you will most likely be able to lower them with lifestyle changes. Later, in Chapters 2 and 3, I will discuss how you can modify your cholesterol levels with behavioral changes such as exercise and nutrition. If you are in the High Risk range, try behavioral changes first. However, if your blood tests don't improve, be prepared to take medication.

Risk 4: High Blood Pressure

Risk number four is High Blood Pressure, or Hypertension. When we talk about hypertension, we look at two numbers called the systolic (the higher number) and diastolic (the lower number). Generally, we rely on the lower diastolic number to define hypertension.

Over time, high blood pressure stresses the lining of our arteries and creates a site for plaque to begin to build up. This was the early basis for defining this process as "hardening" of the arteries. The "stiffer" the wall of the artery, the less give it has as the heart forces blood out into the circulatory system. The pressure inside a stiff, hardened blood vessel is much higher than inside a soft pliable vessel. Unfortunately, people often overlook the fact that the only way to determine their blood pressure is to have it taken with a blood pressure monitoring device.

The Importance of Taking Your Blood Pressure

I am reminded of a time when a man in his forties came in to our Emergency Department complaining of a slight headache and a little shortness of breath while mowing his lawn. Since he exhibited no other symptoms, and his condition seemed stable, there was no rush for me to see him. However, when the nurse found that his blood pressure was 240/140 mmHg, she immediately alerted me, and we ended up treating him as an acute, hypertensive emergency, saving him from a certain catastrophe!

To be normal, your blood pressure should remain below 160/90 mmHg, but always check with your doctor. There are many variables in defining a "normal" blood pressure, as indicated in Table 1.1.

Risk 5: Diabetes Mellitus

Risk number five is Diabetes Mellitus. There are two types of Diabetes, the inherited Type I (Juvenile diabetes) and Type II (Adult Onset diabetes). The inherited type requires insulin shots and, unfortunately, leads to early aging which is a high risk for heart disease. For best control, this condition must be managed with your doctor.

Surprisingly, Type II diabetics often have more insulin in their blood than normal people do. For some reason, their insulin doesn't get to the cells or isn't as effective once it does. Furthermore, the cause of this kind of diabetes is much more than just a sugar problem; it also involves fats, proteins and minerals. Diabetes is a complicated disease that affects your tiniest blood vessels, including those of your brain, heart, eyes and kidneys. The consequences are similar to those of atherosclerosis in that blood can't get nutrients to the cells. Thus, diffuse disease occurs in all organs, including the heart, and eventually leads to an early heart attack. Having a complicated metabolic course, though, doesn't mean you can't change your behavior at the Point PM on the Health Continuum to prolong your life. It turns out that Type II diabetics respond incredibly well to proper nutrition and exercise.

Risk 6: Physical Inactivity

NOTE:

"Before supper walk a little; after supper do the same."

Desadenus
Erasmus,
1466-1536

Physical Inactivity is risk number six. Numerous investigations have reported that increased physical activity protects against coronary artery disease. One study in particular showed that the risk for heart disease is cut in half with 2,000+ Calories of additional physical exertion per week.[7] There are probably a lot of reasons why this occurs since exercise interacts with so many other mechanisms that lead to a reduced risk for heart attacks.

For example, here are just a few of the protective effects of exercise:

1. Lowers blood pressure.
2. Decreases heart rate.
3. Helps to control obesity.
4. Improves lipid profile.
5. Diminishes glucose intolerance.

6. Strengthens the heart muscle.

7. Maintains a steady heart rhythm.

8. Protects against the outpouring of adrenaline associated with stress.

9. Drains extra fluid away from tissues.

As you will see later in this book, there are many more benefits from exercise.

The Minor Risks

Risk 7: Obesity

Obesity, risk number seven, is unequivocally associated with a higher incidence of death from heart disease. In addition, obesity is a risk for interruptions in the rhythm of the heart beat. As you will learn in Chapter 2, "Physical Fitness," it is difficult to define obesity since there are so many different methods to assess the body's composition.

One study suggests that obesity has such a high independent relationship with heart disease that it should be considered a major risk factor, not a minor one.[8] This study is believable if you imagine the tremendous strain on the heart to pump blood through 25, or sometimes even 100 extra pounds of unneeded fat. For example, imagine lugging around a 55 pound bag of dog food all day. The heart has to speed up, as well as contract stronger to force blood through all this extra tissue. One of the striking abnormal vital signs I see with obese people is that their fast heart rate invariably comes down with weight loss. But, like any pump, the heart will give out if constantly overworked and strained.

NOTE:
One study suggests that obesity . . . should be considered a major risk factor. . .

Another link obesity has with heart disease is that fat infiltrates the heart muscle causing rhythm interruptions which could actually lead to the most serious of rhythm disturbances, called ventricular fibrillation. This phenomena leaves the ventricles of the heart literally quivering without any heartbeat or pumping action. The result is sudden death!

Risk 8: Psychological Stress

Risk eight is Psychological Stress. Actually, the risk is not the stress itself but the way in which you handle it. The manifestation of stress has been classified as the Type A or Type B personality. The Type A personality is characterized as one who is impatient, driven and competitive; the Type B personality assumes a more laid back, easy going, take-it-as-you-go nature.

NOTE: *... the risk is not the stress itself but the way in which you handle it.*

The Type A personality can further be subdivided into two kinds . . . productive and potentially destructive. Productive Type A's channel their stress into enthusiastic and healthy behaviors. They have learned how to externalize their feelings and communicate their emotions as a way of managing their stress. Destructive Type A's internalize their emotions, producing pent up anger and hostility which adversely impacts on their health.

Our nervous and endocrine systems were designed to help us deal with stress. In fact, initially both systems release the same biological chemical, adrenaline, to help our bodies prepare for the "fight or flight" response. We even have a long-term stress management system controlled by our adrenal glands. When there are too many acute demands or too long a chronic demand on these systems, our bodies wear out. We develop internal ulcers, a compromised immune system; or metabolic abnormalities, all of which lead to cardiac stress and deterioration.

Risk 9: Age

The last risk factor, Age, is unquestionably associated with an increased incidence of heart disease. After all, age is progressive and the older we get the more likely disease is to occur. Since age is not a factor you can control, then why should it be considered as a manageable risk? The answer is, that in addition to chronological age, there is biological age. How may times have you heard, "Oh, he's a young fifty year old." Your life style affects your biological age. If you happen to have a strong constitution but have not yet paid the price of poor health behaviors, eventually you will! This is as inevitable as the sun coming up each day.

NOTE:
Your life style affects your biological age.

Generally for men, the price is paid during what I call the "decay decade" of their forties. A case in point occurred just the other day when a 48 year old man dragged into the office, plopped down on the sofa and said, "I'm sick and tired of being <u>sick</u> and <u>tired</u>!" He went on, "My body just can't keep up with my mind any more."

Women go through the "decay decade" during menopause. Their bodies change. For example, heart disease kills the greatest number of men above the age of forty, for women, it's after menopause.

You can start now, however, to prepare to pay a far lower price . . . by making a transition to positive life styles that will prolong and improve your health.

How to Change

NOTE:
. . . You can
permanently
change or control
seven of the nine
risks to your
health.

For many people in search of a quick fix, the easy way out is to take medication. However, by popping pills we pay the price of side effects and isolated treatment of single issues. This compartmentalized approach ignores the holistic concept of our essence . . . total well being. In other words, a pill may reduce your cholesterol, but what about your weight or the fat in your blood vessels and heart muscle? Drugs may alleviate indigestion, but that is only temporary because it ignores the underlying cause of the problem. Furthermore, we frequently "burn out" on these medications.

The band aid approach is just that . . . cover up your symptoms and let the underlying causes eat away at your very being. Address those underlying causes, and you're well on your way to a healthier, more enjoyable life.

For example, you can **permanently** change or control seven of the nine risk factors:

Cigarette Smoking
Total Blood Cholesterol
High Blood Pressure
Diabetes Mellitus, Type II
Physical Inactivity
Obesity
Psychological Stress

By doing so, you will minimize the impact of your family history and age, as I've already discussed. Not only that, but with common sense and simple changes in your lifestyle through exercise, nutrition and stress management, you can profoundly impact on all those risks. Furthermore, we don't have to be drastic all at once; we can make slow reasonable changes. There's just one question. How do we approach the way we live to make specific changes in our lives? The answer is to apply the model of total well being.

Total Well Being

I define total well being as a <u>balanced</u> <u>integration</u> of BODY, MIND and SPIRIT. This is best represented by the model in Figure 1.8.

NOTE:
. . . entry into or focus on one of the areas of Total Well Being leads to change in the other two areas.

Figure 1.8
TOTAL WELL BEING

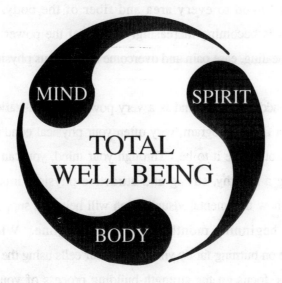

Notice how each component is separate, yet interrelated. Also notice that Total Well Being lies in the center, which represents the connection and integration of all three components. Furthermore, I have personally experienced and have observed in hundreds of patients that entry into or focus on one of the areas leads to what I call "The Movement."

That is, change in one area always involves some movement or change in the other two areas. As you improve your lifestyle behaviors, there is gradually more and more integration of all the areas until you experience total well being. The purpose of this book is to help you begin this movement.

The Mind

There is no doubt that the mental component of total well being is crucial. For years, general practitioners have known that up to eighty percent of their patients' symptoms are psychosomatic. The mind is intricately linked to every area and fiber of the body. The medical community is becoming increasingly aware of the power of the mind to effectuate healing, ease pain and overcome tremendous physical obstacles.

In addition, the mind is a very powerful visualization tool. When you begin a fitness program, very often your physical condition is far from what you would like it to be. Through your mind, you can concentrate on developing a healthy, strong and attractive physical image. You'll be amazed at how this mental visualization will help and support you through the tough beginning months of a fitness regime. When you walk, concentrate on burning fat by visualizing your cells using the fat. When you lift weights, focus on the strength-building process of your muscles. As your body grows stronger, so will your mental prowess through increased energy levels, greater concentration abilities and higher creativity.

The dilemma I face as a health care provider, and you as a consumer, is that the mental arena is so cluttered with conflicting advice and differing approaches that the whole field is confusing. For example, to alleviate your mental stress you can find solutions ranging from psychoanalysis, psychotherapy, behaviorism, humanism, gestalt, biofeedback, transactional analysis, a walk on the beach, meditation, yoga, acupuncture and many more. Even though I have personally explored many of these solutions, I have no idea which one is best for you. I am convinced, however, that one or more of these techniques is right for you. Since this is so important to behavioral change, I will discuss it in more depth in Chapter 4.

The Spirit

Next, consider the component of spirit or soul. No one could question the importance or influence of spirituality throughout human history. Yet, the spiritual community is also filled with many different philosophies, religions and beliefs. Just think of the various religions with all their denominations and sects. What about all the new age philosophies, spiritual retreats, gurus and self-empowerment programs? Again, I know there is one or more approach that is best for you, but how do those of us in the healing arts, or for that matter how does anyone, truly know the solution to another person's spiritual needs?

> **NOTE:**
> *"If the head and the body are to be well, you must begin by curing the soul."*
>
> Plato,
> 427-347 B.C.

For purposes of this book, I look upon the spirit as energy . . . the energy needed to make the movement toward Total Well Being . . . the energy to change. One way to initiate that change is through trust in a power greater than ourselves. This does not take away our responsibility to take action. However, it does make decisions easier because our interest changes from control for self to self control for a higher purpose.

The very nature of spiritual development is nebulous and unstructured. The importance of the spirit is to help you reach a contentment level in all the phases of your life. There are a multitude of opportunities for your mind and your spirit to grow and change. These growth opportunities will present themselves to you throughout your life. Fitness will help you to bring about contentment and peace of mind through the building of your spirit. This brings us to our physical nature where there are specific and objective methods to help people promote better physical well being.

The Body

NOTE:

the benefits of exercise will impact on the functioning of your body's biochemistry, physiology and anatomy . . . your life!

Physical wellness or fitness consists of four elements: Body Composition, Flexibility, Strength and Aerobics. Body composition results from that which we ingest or inhale. We can be very specific about recommendations for improved nutrition. Furthermore, I can give you specific, no-nonsense techniques to quantitatively assess and analyze your physical nature. Then, from this objective data, you can be given formulas to create your own prescription to improve your physical fitness.

Unlike the mind and spirit, there isn't much confusion about what we need to do in order to make changes in our lives regarding our bodies. I think this approach is also the most effective and efficient for people in our industrialized, highly technological society which forces us to function mainly from the left-brain. This means that we are more comfortable with straightforward, objective, numbers-oriented approaches to change. Thus, I suggest that the physical component, the body, is the most reasonable entry point into the model of total well being.

I know that the most valuable benefits you will get from exercise include improvements in how you look, feel and act. But more profoundly, the benefits of exercise will impact on the functioning of your body's biochemistry, physiology and anatomy . . . your life! You will see how in the following chapter.

SUMMARY

We <u>can</u> live a long, happy, healthy life, and we intuitively, if not factually, know how to do it. To be sure, our society places enormous external pressures on us that compromise our lifestyles so we develop unwellness, disease and, often, an untimely death. Our modern health care system is designed to effectively help us deal with disease but places little emphasis on prevention. Fortunately, we have the power within us to change the way we live and interrupt that slow march toward degenerative diseases; indeed, to create total well being.

One way to learn what new behavior patterns we need to adopt is to look at the major causes of death among us today. Clearly, it boils down to one thing . . . plaque build-up in our blood vessels . . . atherosclerosis. The cells in our bodies are totally dependent on oxygen and other nutrients carried to them in the blood stream. Compromised blood flow from plaque build-up diminishes the cellular function leading to unwellness and disease, particularly heart attack and stroke.

There are at least nine risk factors associated with the development of atherosclerosis: Positive Family History, Cigarette Smoking, Elevated Blood Cholesterol Levels, High Blood Pressure, Diabetes Mellitus, Physical Inactivity, Obesity, Psychological Stress and Age. With lifestyle changes, we can definitely and permanently control <u>seven</u> of these risk factors!

One way to identify approaches that will help us control these risks is by looking at the model of total well being which is defined as an <u>integrated</u> <u>balance</u> of Body, Mind and Spirit. The mind and spirit components of this model contain a variety of approaches, techniques and philosophies which are often nebulous, untried or foreign to our nature.

Despite this, there are one or more approaches that will work specifically for you. On the other hand, entry into this model through our bodies by physical fitness and nutrition can be accomplished with straight-forward, objective, no-nonsense formulae.

Resources

The following books and monograph provide a historical account which helps put in perspective the way our health care system evolved over the years. Hepner's book, **The Healthy Strategy Game**, approaches it from the standpoint of management and, therefore, his book is "must reading" for anyone who contemplates becoming a health executive (1).

Illich, in **Medical Nemisis**, unravels the morass of our "Iatrogenic" epidemic (iatros = physician and genic = origin); our physician induced crisis (2). So often, I hear people blame doctors as our medical nemesis. Illich, however, points out that lay people have the power to take control of our medicalized industrial complex. Is he saying that blame is a subterfuge for shirking ones own responsibility?

Dr. Annis, in **Code Blue, Health Care Crisis**, argues that what our society declares as a health care crisis is really a crisis in government (3). And, rather than accept the reforms being bantered about by our political system, we should reject them as government intrusion, which only compounds the problem. Interestingly enough, this cry resembles that being heard by natural healers who deplore the Food and Drug Administration's designs on controlling the health food industry. Does alternative medicine and orthodox medicine have something in common . . . have we come full circle? Do we, as individuals, have the wisdom, and can we take the power back into our own hands to regain a free health care society?

The plan proposed by The National Center for Policy Analysis, *An Agenda for Solving America's Health Care Crisis*, gives us an <u>excellent</u> framework for change (4). This plan was created by a multi-disciplinary task force free from special interest groups; therefore, it takes emotion and bias out of the equation. It is clear, concise and excellent reading for everyone. Whatever your persuasion, the additional knowledge that you will gain from these resources will greatly contribute to a more thoughtful and ultimately successful conclusion to serve the health care needs in the future.

My patients frequently ask if they should see an alternative health care provider. I do not hesitate to say yes, if they have been thoroughly evaluated by an orthodox medical practitioner, and they meet these three criteria:

1. Orthodox medicine has provided a diagnosis but has no curative treatment.
2. Orthodox treatment is not successful.
3. They want a "third" opinion.

I am coming to believe that a fourth criterion should be included. That is, we should follow what we believe in our heart of hearts. I am beginning to realize that our inner-held beliefs are more powerful and, therefore, more effective than any external influence.

In this day and age with the incredulous and dynamic flux taking place in modern medicine, we physicians are opening up to preventive medicine by considering many types of alternative health care. Perhaps a better phrase would be complementary health care. Fortunately, many credible and capable physicians have formed groups to support one another and share in their knowledge, experience and research to promote better health care for their patients and the nation.

Contact your local county medical association or any of following three organizations. The American Holistic Medical Association emphasizes the whole person, physical, mental, emotional and spiritual (5). The American College for Advancement in Medicine emphasizes the practice of nutritional supplementation and intravenous vitamin and chelation therapy (6). The Physicians Committee for Responsible Medicine promotes preventive medicine through innovative nutritional programs and opposes human and animal experimentation (7). These organizations will provide you with literature, references and referrals.

2 PHYSICAL FITNESS

Introduction

I believe that people in our left-brain, numbers-oriented, objective society are more likely to enter the model of total well being through physical fitness than through either the mental or spiritual pathways. As I discussed in Chapter 1, the body, mind and spirit are interconnected; therefore, improvements in one area enable us to experience benefits in the other two areas. Most of us know from some experience, if not intuitively, that with exercise we simply <u>feel</u> <u>better</u>. In fact, feeling better, looking better and having positive feedback from those around us, are our strongest motivating factors. However, there are a host of other benefits to be gained from following a fitness program. Knowing about these benefits may create additional motivation for you to get started and maintain a daily exercise routine. That is what I want you to do. Let's begin by answering the question, "What is physical fitness?"

NOTE:
"A vigorous five-mile walk will do more for an unhappy man but otherwise healthy adult than all the medicine in the world."

Paul Dudley White, M.D. 1886-1973

What is Physical Fitness?

Physical fitness is a combination of Body Composition, Flexibility, Strength, and Aerobics. Just like the model for total well being, physical fitness also consists of an <u>integrated</u> <u>balance</u> of all components, Figure 2.1.

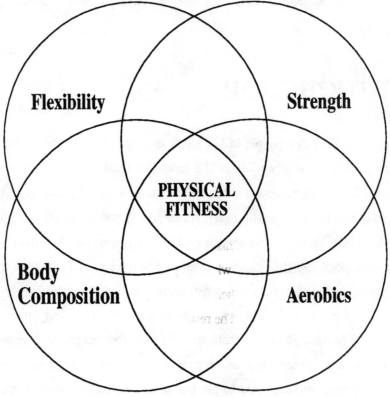

Figure 2.1
THE MODEL FOR PHYSICAL FITNESS

Balanced Integration

Each component is unique since you can derive its benefits only from doing activities particular to that component. In fact, if you focus on just one activity, you may miss out on the benefits you would gain from doing activities in the other components. For instance, I have known yoga instructors with phenomenal flexibility who had to relearn how to walk or jog properly in order to build up their aerobic capacity. I have treated body builders with "award winning biceps" whose cholesterol counts were sky high . . . a set up for atherosclerosis.

No matter how dedicated a person is to one component of the model, the only real path to total well being is to integrate and balance all of the components. That is, the sum of the parts is greater than the whole. Following a balanced, integrated routine will yield anatomical, physiological and biochemical benefits that go way beyond those you would receive from less scientific, exercise plans.

Exercise Promotes Life

Pause for a moment and reflect on all of the benefits that you already know result from exercise. Did you consider one of the most important . . . prolonged life? This benefit was actually proven in 1993 and reported by Paffenbarger, et. al. when they followed the histories of 16,936 Harvard alumni and compared their ages at death to their levels of physical activity throughout their lives.[1] The results showed that those who expended 2,000+ additional Calories of activity on a weekly basis prolonged their lives by an average of two and one half years. This equates to approximately 20 miles of walking or jogging per week. However, you can benefit from only a small amount of activity over and beyond a sedentary lifestyle. For example, burning only 1,000 additional Calories per week would include such activities as parking your car so you would be forced to walk a few extra blocks to work, walking up a few flights of stairs each day, taking a lunch time stroll, gardening or engaging in leisure time sports.

NOTE:
. . . you can benefit from only a small amount of activity over and beyond a sedentary lifestyle.

This may not seem like a worthwhile number of extra years to some of you but remember, these numbers are just averages. There were many in this study who lived a lot longer. And so far, we've been referring only to the quantity of life; what about the quality?

Quality-versus-Quantity

Even though quality is more difficult to measure, it's more profound in its implications. Quality is a subjective assessment and, therefore, doesn't yield the objective information science requires to statistically prove a point. However, the literature abounds with studies showing that people in wellness programs have greater productivity, less illness and lead happier personal lives.[2,3,4]

Listen to Your Body

NOTE:

"All the soarings of my mind begin in my blood."

Rainer Maria Rilke, 1921

Improved physical fitness can reduce all of the risk factors associated with the leading causes of illness and death. Exercise does enable us to live better and longer. However, it can only do this if we listen to our bodies. Each of us has his or her own set of connections between the body and the mind . . . a set of harmonies, if you will . . . that continually communicate our physicalness to us.

As you begin to exercise on a regular basis, you will be conditioning not only your body, but also your mind and spirit. In so doing, your intuition will become more and more sensitive to the messages your body is sending. The connection between mind and body will become stronger as you propel yourself toward total well being. As your body becomes stronger, so will you develop your ability to listen to it.

Thus, when considering total well being, we need to understand how the slow progressive degenerative diseases impact longevity, and how we can intervene through exercise. However, before starting to modify our lifestyles through a physical fitness plan designed to implement long term intervention, we also need to understand the relationship between exercise and the potential for its dire consequence . . . sudden death.

Sudden Death

The exact cause of sudden death is unknown. After all, how could scientists design a safe double blind study to test the causes of sudden death? I can't imagine who would volunteer for the experimental group. We hypothesize that sudden death occurs when the blood vessels feeding the heart are blocked and the heart muscle doesn't get enough oxygen delivered to it. In young people this is because the arteries that feed the heart are anatomically abnormal or because the heart muscle obstructs blood flow to the muscle cells.[5] In people who are 30 years and older, it almost always is due to atherosclerosis in the arteries that feed the heart muscle cells.[6] As the heart muscle becomes exhausted, the cells trigger extra beats which move closer and closer together. This process finally produces such a rapid beating of the heart that it can't keep up and simply stops . . . sudden death.

NOTE: *. . . when one examines the data . . . heart attacks and sudden death occur with a much higher incidence in people who are sedentary . . .*

The press brought sudden death to the public's attention when they overreacted to the deaths of people like Jim Fix by so distorting the facts that many people are convinced that any type of strenuous exercise will lead to instant death, regardless of age. More recently, headlines proclaimed such statements as "Exercise Linked To Death" which were based upon two 1994 studies reporting a positive relationship between heart attacks and exercise.[7,8] However, when one examines the data hidden in these reports, the studies actually prove that heart attacks and sudden death occur with a much higher incidence in people who are <u>sedentary</u> and do very little exercise.

The truth is that the benefits of physical fitness far outweigh the tiny chance of exercise induced "sudden death." To begin with, as mentioned above, anyone over the age of 30 who dies during exercise does so because of atherosclerosis which, itself, can be prevented with exercise. However, think about this subtle but extremely important fact . . . a fact that cannot be adequately evaluated in retrospective studies such as those cited above. Were the people who died of sudden death during physical activity exercising <u>properly</u> and, therefore, <u>safely</u>? For example, did they undergo proper medical clearance? Were they warmed up? Were they properly hydrated? Did they exercise within a safe training heart rate zone? I strongly suspect that those few people who died violated proper exercise rules. And, if they had followed those rules, the small incidence of exercise related "sudden death" would probably have vanished. This is one of the main reasons I wrote this book and its companion manual on exercise, so you could realize the benefits of improved fitness by exercising properly <u>and</u> safely.

Now, let's look at the individual components of physical fitness and see how each works to help us achieve total well being.

Body Composition

In addition to exercise, body composition results from the following components: Nutrition, Ingestants and Inhalants, Figure 2.2.

Figure 2.2
THE COMPONENTS OF BODY COMPOSITION

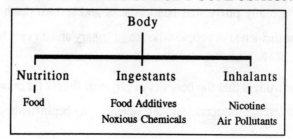

Nutrition refers to the food substances that we take in, such as carbohydrates, proteins, fats, vitamins, minerals and water. Ingestants include all those additives in our food chain, plus noxious chemicals such as caffeine, alcohol and drugs. Drugs that affect us may be over the counter, prescription medications or illegal drugs. Inhalants include nicotine and a host of environmental air pollutants. For now, suffice it to say that all of these components, whether taken into your system directly or indirectly, affect our bodies' composition. In Chapter 3, "Nutrition," I will explain how these components impact on your total well being, because we truly are what we eat.

When most people think about body composition, they focus on the measurements we use to determine our bodies' composition. The first thing that comes to mind is the most readily available measurement - total body weight.

Total Body Weight

Unfortunately, total body weight is the most unreliable measure of body composition. Compare two people of the same age and height who each weigh 200 pounds. One is a strong fit athlete and the other is an unconditioned couch potato. You probably picture the athlete as firm, muscular and healthy looking, while you imagine the couch potato as round and flabby with a pasty pallor. Both, however, have the same total body weight. This shows how misleading measuring body weight alone can be. This is especially true if we want to use body composition as an indication of our health status.

NOTE:
. . . total body weight is the most unreliable measure of bod composition.

Body Water

The main reason total body weight is unreliable is because of the amount of water in our body. Over 70% of our weight is water which is very heavy compared to other body tissues, and it fluctuates rapidly with our intake and output. For example, exercising in hot, humid weather or in rubberized suits causes marked water loss through sweat. The resulting weight loss is strictly artificial, however, since it will be put back on as soon as you rehydrate through normal eating and drinking.

Another variable occurs with strenuous exercise. This causes muscles to retain water, resulting in a transient weight gain. Frequently, patients come in after a week of heavy exercise only to find that they gained, rather than lost, weight. It's the water retention in their muscles that gives this false information. They make up for it in the long run, but they need to gauge their progress by taking average weights over a longer period of time.

Total body weight may also give false information when it comes to "dieting." Much of our body water is bound up by cells. When we decrease caloric intake and use up fat from our cells they shrink and release water which is eliminated though our kidneys. This water loss occurs rapidly at first, then slows down. Remember the last time you went on a diet and, in the beginning, lost a lot of weight and then gradually your weight loss slowed down? Initially, you were simply losing water, not fat.

Body Weight and Exercise

Total body weight can also give misleading information relative to your fitness training. For example, let's look at the results from the participants in our Institute. These data, and those I'll refer to throughout this chapter, were taken from over 500 adults who took part in a supervised exercise program for three months. They were tested before and after the program. The data were statistically analyzed, and I'll simply use the word "significant" to indicate statistically significant changes that resulted. Furthermore, I've calculated the % change* that occurred over the three months to give you a better indication of the magnitude of improvement. The body weight changes shown in Table 2.1 are very informative.

Notice that there was an average weight loss of only two pounds. However, the measurement of their % body fat decreased by 3%, representing a significant 10.4% change. With this loss in body fat, their fat weight significantly decreased and their lean body mass, mostly muscle, significantly increased.

These results help explain why total body weight doesn't change much with exercise. Muscle weighs a lot more than fat because muscle cells contain so much more water than fat cells. Remember, oil (fat cells) and water don't mix. Therefore, the <u>increase</u> in muscle mass with a <u>decrease</u> in body fat leaves a net result of little or no change in total body weight.

NOTE:
. . . the <u>increase</u> in muscle mass with a <u>decrease</u> in body fat leaves a net result of little or no change in total body weight.

Table 2.1
IMPROVEMENTS IN BODY COMPOSITION

	Averages		
	Before	After	% Change
Total Weight	177 lbs	175 lbs	-1.1%
% Body Fat	28.8%	25.8 %	-10.4%
Fat Weight	51 lbs	45 lbs	-11.8%
Lean Weight	126 lbs	130 lbs	+3.2%

* % Change = (After - Before) ÷ Before x 100. For example, if a number changes from 10 to 12, that represents a 20% increase.

However, participants reported that their clothes fit looser, and their friends told them how much better they looked and asked how much weight they had lost.

I continually tell my patients who want to lose weight to forget striving for some magic number. Instead, define your goal as whatever your weight is when:

1. You feel great.
2. You think you look great.
3. You think others think you look great!

Percentage of Body Fat

NOTE:
. . . the best measure of body composition is the determination of your percentage of body fat.

By far, the best measure of body composition is the determination of your percentage of body fat. This measure adjusts for the fluctuations of your total body water. Unfortunately, accurate and reliable measurements require expensive equipment and/or well trained personnel. You may wish to visit any health or fitness organization (health club, university or hospital) where they will test your body fat for you. Or, obtain a copy of the companion manual to this book (1) where I will teach you how to measure your own body fat plus the other measures of body composition discussed on the next page.

Body Mass Index

Body mass index is another way to determine your body composition. This measure takes your body's surface area into consideration which, to some extent, compensates for the big muscular - versus - the big fat person. Moreover, this index is frequently used in medical population studies, so there are many health statistics relating to this index.

Anthropometric Measurements

There is another way to assess your body composition, commonly used by body builders, which is called anthropometric measurements. This involves measuring the circumference of the parts of your body that you want to test, for example, your abdomen, torso, arms and legs. This is also known as girth measurement. For the <u>average</u> <u>person</u> interested in all around fitness training, these measurements don't change much.

For example, as shown in Table 2.2, our participants did not significantly change their girth measurements except for a small, but significant decrease of one inch around their waists. The reason for the lack of changes in other parts of their bodies, including their chests and extremities, is probably due to their increase in muscular development which was off set by their loss in fat tissue. Therefore, the net circumferential measurement did not change significantly.

NOTE:
For the <u>average</u> <u>person</u>... circumference measurements don't change much.

Table 2.2
CHANGES IN ANTHROPOMETRIC MEASUREMENTS

| | Average Inches | | |
	Before	After	% Change
Waist	35.5	34.5	- 1.0
Chest	39.8	39.4	- 0.4
Thigh	22.7	22.3	- 0.4
Calf	14.7	14.8	+ 0.1
Forearm	10.6	10.5	- 0.1
Upper Arm	12.0	12.1	+ 0.1

However, the fact that their waist sizes decreased by an average of one inch is important, not only because of their looks, but because it has recently been discovered that the waist to hip ratio is a number that can predict the incidence of heart attacks!

Waist to Hip Ratio

NOTE:
To decrease your risk for heart disease. . . you would rather be more like the "pear" shape . . . than the "apple" shape.

There is a significant relationship between your waist and hip size called the waist to hip ratio. This is determined by dividing your waist circumference by your hip circumference. The larger your abdomen in relation to your hips, the greater your association with high cholesterol, hypertension, heart disease and diabetes.[9,10] In other words, you would rather be more like the "pear" shape, less fat around your waist than your hips, than the "apple" shape with a bigger abdomen.

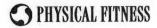

Determine Your Waist to Hip Ratio

This is such an important indication of our health status that we are beginning to perform this measurement on all of our participants in the Institute. I recommend you make this determination on yourself. First, measure your waist size at your belly button and round it off to quarters of an inch, e.g. 36.00, 36.25, 36.50, or 36.75 inches and record it below.

Waist Size [ ] inches

Then, measure your hip circumference around your buttocks where you are the widest.

Hip Size [ ] inches

Next, you are going to divide your <u>waist</u> measurement by your <u>hip</u> measurement to get the ratio.

For example, I measure exactly 36 inches around my waist and 40 1/4 inches around my hips. My ratio is calculated as follows:

$$\frac{\text{Waist Size in inches} = 36.00}{\text{Hip Size in inches} = 40.25} = \text{Ratio of } .89$$

Notice that you want the numerator (waist size) to be low and the denominator (hip size) to be <u>relatively</u> higher. Therefore, what kind of a number do you want for the ratio . . . high or low? You want a low number. In this case the further below one the better.

So, go ahead with your measurements:

Waist Size in inches = ▮

Hip Size in inches = ▮

= Ratio of ▮

Compare your ratio with the following standards:

		Ratio	
	Ideal	Moderate Risk	High Risk
Men	<	1.0	>
Women	<	.85	>

For men, your ratio should be less than 1.0 . . . if less than 1.0, you have no risk associated with those conditions mentioned above . . . the higher your ratio above 1.0, the greater your risk.

For women, your ratio should be less than 0.85 . . . the higher your ratio the greater your risk. Notice, women should have a lower ratio to compensate for the natural deposition of adipose (fat) tissue around their hips (higher denominator).

Now, if you go back to the data from our participants in Table 2.2, it shows that a general fitness training program can be beneficial for your health since there is a decrease in waist size with presumably no increase in hip measurement.

Flexibility

Flexibility is one of the most important components of physical fitness. And, you improve your flexibility only by stretching. Since this is so often forgotten and underrated in the field of exercise, I put stretching before strengthening and aerobic training in all my fitness assessment and instruction programs. There are two health reasons why flexibility is so important.

Stretching Prevents Injury

To begin with, you should know that the best way to prevent injury is to stretch before and after you exercise. Injury is the number one cause of drop out from exercise programs. Therefore, preventing injury from happening will eliminate one of the most tempting excuses to quit exercise. Injury is such a good excuse because it can be a legitimate reason to put off exercise. However, as so many have found out, once you've put your exercise program on hold, it's easy to continue putting it off until you drop it altogether.

> **NOTE:**
> *. . . the best way to prevent injury is to stretch before and after you exercise.*

Stretching Prevents Low Back Pain

The second reason stretching is important is because increased flexibility decreases the risk factor for low back pain syndrome . . . a condition that affects over 80% of our population. In fact, the diagnosis and treatment of low back pain accounts for the greatest expense in workman's compensation costs, not to mention the agony suffered by millions of Americans.

Proper stretching and strengthening of your abdominal muscles, the muscles in back of your thighs (the hamstrings) and your buttocks combine to markedly decrease the incidence and severity of low back pain syndrome. Indeed, many orthopedic surgeons send their patients through our program at the Institute to reduce the necessity for back surgery with remarkable, lasting success. Generally, our patients report that they have decreased bouts of back pain after the program and less severity of pain with the episodes they do have. Much of this is due to their improved stretching ability.

For example, look at the improvements in their flexibility in Table 2.3. These measurements were obtained with the standard sit and reach test which is performed by sitting and reaching forward over a specially designed box and measuring the distance reached in inches. Initially, women are more flexible than men by four inches. After three months in the program, however, both men and women significantly increase their flexibility by about one and one half inches.

Table 2.3
IMPROVEMENTS IN FLEXIBILITY

	Average Inches		
	Before	After	% Change
Female	15.4	16.9	+ 9.7%
Male	11.4	13.0	+ 14.0%

Of course, you don't really need to do any tests to know that your flexibility improves with stretching. Gradually, it becomes easier to get in and out of your car, to reach for things in your closet, to enjoy your recreational activities . . . to simply move!

Strength Training

You will derive numerous benefits from strength training. Perhaps the most significant, although not immediately obvious, has to do with weight loss. In fact, many of the more progressive weight loss programs are turning to strength training before aerobic activity in order to help facilitate weight loss and maintenance. There are metabolic reasons for this.

NOTE:

. . . weight loss programs are turning to strength training . . . to help facilitate weight loss and maintenance.

Weight Loss

Muscle tissue has high metabolic demands. Therefore, it uses considerably more calories to simply maintain itself. This is especially true when you compare muscle cells to fat cells. Therefore, when you combine strength training with a proper diet, an additive effect occurs. As your body composition changes by increasing lean muscle mass and decreasing fat, your metabolic rate increases and consumes even more calories. Assuming that you continue your proper nutrition and exercise routine, the pounds will literally melt off!

Improvements in Strength

There is no question that you will gain strength in your entire body with proper exercise. Just look at the increased strength of our participants after only three months in the program, Table 2.4. Both men and women significantly improved their upper and low body strength as measured on a special hydraulic strength measuring device. Their gains in strength were consistent in all muscle groups. This supports what I said earlier about how exercise increases muscle mass, or lean body weight.

Table 2.4
IMPROVEMENTS IN MUSCLE STRENGTH

Average Strength in Pressure Pounds Measured on a Special Hydraulic Press		
	BEFORE	AFTER
Pectoralis Front of chest	164	179
Trapezius Back of neck	131	149
Deltoid Top of shoulder	84	95
Latissimus Sides of chest	134	146
Quadriceps Front of thigh	131	151
Hamstrings Back of thigh	71	84

Naturally, women are not as strong as men in absolute terms, but, based upon a % increase in strength, women improved as much as the men, Table 2.5. For example, on a relative basis, women improved more in the pectoralis, deltoid and hamstring muscles while men improved more in the other muscle groups. It's not important what muscle groups improved in which sex, rather that women can derive the same benefits from strength training as men.

Table 2.5
% INCREASE IN STRENGTH

Muscle Group	Men	Women
Pectoralis	9.0	11.7
Trapezius	14.8	14.0
Deltoid	14.3	14.6
Latissimus	10.6	7.1
Quadriceps	16.2	15.6
Hamstrings	16.9	18.2

Perhaps the most important advantage to strength training is how much better you will look. This is especially true if you build muscles to fill up the spaces under your skin vacated by the loss of fat. You will also move better with the combination of increased strength and improved flexibility. But there are other benefits as well. For instance, as you are able to move your body more easily, you'll have more fun doing the recreational activities you enjoy or playing with your children or grandchildren. You'll also cut down on your potential for injury as you strengthen the connective tissue associated with your muscles and bones.

Always remember that strength development is a unique component of physical fitness. The only way to derive its benefits is to incorporate strength training into your exercise program. And as you do, listen to your body. As you listen, you will become more and more engaged with your physical self and, thus, more self-aware. You will be moving even closer to total well being, and you will feel great!

Aerobics

Aerobic activity is defined as any activity that increases and sustains your heart rate over a given period of time.

From working with hundreds of patients, it has become apparent to me that the concept of a sustained heart rate needs to be re-emphasized. Again and again, after discussing the importance of exercise with my patients, especially those who have risk factors for heart disease, they respond by saying they will take up some leisure sport. Although this is better than nothing and may be a good beginning, leisure sports do not provide the full benefits equivalent to true aerobic activity. Only through sustained aerobic activity will your body switch from burning carbohydrates to burning fat. The best aerobic activity is one that you can sustain at a moderate level of exertion for a 20 to 30 minute period. Sustain is the key word here; the longer you can sustain the aerobic level the more fat you will burn. As you will see, a stop and go sport such as tennis will not burn fat.

A Leisure Sport: Tennis

I began playing tennis in my thirties. In the beginning, I carried only the necessary two balls during my turn at serve. It seemed to make the game move along faster. Well, it didn't take me long in the Miami heat to realize that carrying that third ball and hunting it down gave me a legitimate break from exercising! Indeed, I could turn this little foray into a long enough stall to totally catch my breath and cool down. Little did I know at the time that by allowing my heart rate to return toward normal, I was diminishing the aerobic benefit from my exercise. No wonder I didn't lose any weight and couldn't run for any distance when I started jogging.

That's not to say that a competitive style of singles tennis can't be aerobically exhaustive. It's a great game and a lot of fun. But, be honest with yourself and keep a proper perspective regarding your motives for whatever aerobic activity you choose.

True aerobic exercise includes such activities as walking, jogging, bicycling, swimming, rope skipping, calisthenics to music, etc. These exercises use large muscles and are continuous, which sustains your heart rate.

What Happens to Your Body During Aerobic Training

I find that most people are amazed when they discover what goes on in their bodies with aerobic training. Indeed, this whole process is a miracle of life and involves a host of anatomical, physiological and biochemical events. I want to summarize this process hoping that you will be even more inspired to do aerobic exercise once you see how it can contribute so much to your total well being.

NOTE:
The whole process of aerobic training is a miracle of life.

Simply put, aerobic activity involves the capture of oxygen from air, the transportation of oxygen throughout your body and the transfer of oxygen into your muscles. "Bioenergy" is then produced resulting in movement. But, there is much more to it than just that! Follow along with Figure 2.3 to see what I mean.

Step 1:
Your Lungs and the Transport of Oxygen

You inhale air through your nasal/oral cavity, where it then passes into your large airways, and finally through smaller and smaller airways until it reaches millions of tiny air sacs. From there, oxygen, the driving force of life, diffuses across the membranes of your air sacs and tiny blood vessels into your blood stream. At that point, oxygen is ready to be transported by red blood cells throughout your body.

Our brains orchestrate complicated reflexes that control the nerves and muscles of our chests to coordinate our breathing and the movement of air in and out of our lungs. Aerobic exercise improves this entire process, from the coordination of breathing, to the movement of oxygen into our blood streams and the increase in red blood cells to carry more oxygen. And so far, we've only scratched the surface of what goes on with aerobic activity!

Step 2:
Your Cardiovascular System

Next, the cardiovascular system comes into play, which includes your heart and blood vessels. Aerobic training strengthens your heart muscle and improves the electrical conduction in your heart to ensure a strong steady beat. This results in an increased blood flow of oxygen and other nutrients to muscles throughout your body. When oxygen reaches your tiny blood vessels, called capillaries, it diffuses into your muscle cells. Aerobic conditioning greatly increases the number of capillaries in your tissues to improve oxygen delivery. So, the more you exercise aerobically,

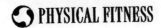

the more oxygen you get to your cells to keep them healthy and functioning properly. This is true for all the cells in your body, which means that aerobic conditioning also improves the function of your nervous, endocrine, gastrointestinal, renal, reproductive, and immunological systems!

Step 3:
The Production of Energy

Once the oxygen diffuses into your muscle cells, specialized structures called mitochondria absorb the oxygen and transform it along a biochemical pathway into bioenergy. This energy causes your muscle fibers to contract, creating movement . . . your goal in exercise. The more you exercise aerobically, the greater your ability to capture oxygen into your cells, and the greater the number of mitochondria to help oxygen produce high levels of bioenergy.

There is More

This is still not the end of the story, however, because there are multiple support systems that assist the capture and movement of oxygen from the air into our muscles to produce the energy we require to live.

For instance, the nervous and endocrine systems control and coordinate this entire process. The nervous system, through an elaborate array of switches and reflexes, immediately controls the rate of our breathing and heartbeat. The endocrine system produces hormones that circulate to various organs and coordinates their functions. Together our nervous and endocrine systems control the stress mechanisms of our bodies. Therefore, as we improve the functioning of these systems with aerobic

NOTE:
. . . there are multiple support systems that assist the capture and movement of oxygen from the air into our muscles to produce the energy we require to live.

activity, we develop an increased capacity to handle stress.

In addition, our gastrointestinal tracts and kidneys function more effectively as greater amounts of oxygen are delivered to their cells. Thus, we absorb nutrients and eliminate waste products more efficiently. This in turn, allows our hearts, lungs and muscles to function more efficiently.

As you can see, therefore, aerobic activity improves the anatomy, physiology and biochemistry of all our systems. Aerobic activity creates a symphony involving the cells, tissues, organs and systems in our bodies, which all work together in balanced harmony to improve our overall well being.

Figure 2.3
THE ANATOMY AND PHYSIOLOGY OF AEROBIC ACTIVITY

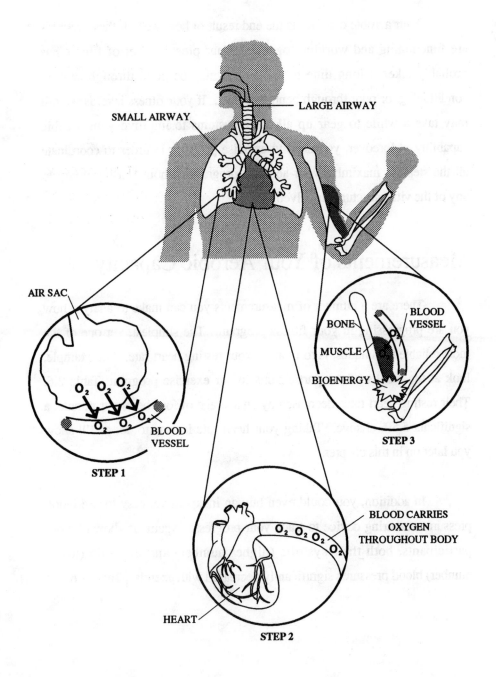

Aerobic Capacity

Your aerobic capacity is the end result of how well all these systems are functioning and working together. Your present level of fitness has probably taken a long time to evolve. It may be good through aerobic conditioning, or poor through benign neglect. If your fitness level is poor, it may take a while to gear up all these systems to improve your aerobic capability. Moreover, you need to exercise properly in order to coordinate all the steps to maximize your aerobics program without causing injury to any of the vital structures involved.

Measurements of Your Aerobic Capacity

There are a number of measurements you can make to analyze how you are progressing in your fitness program. The simplest, yet one of the most reliable techniques, is to monitor your resting heart rate. For example, look at the results of the participants in our exercise program, Table 2.6. Their resting heart rates decreased by an average of four beats per minute, a significant 5.5% change. Taking your heart rate is easy to do, as I'll show you later on in this chapter.

In addition, you could even buy an inexpensive, easy to use blood pressure measuring device to track your progress. Again, as shown by our participants, both their systolic (higher number) and diastolic (lower number) blood pressures significantly decreased with exercise, Table 2.6.

Table 2.6
IMPROVEMENTS IN HEART RATES AND BLOOD PRESSURES

	Averages		
	Before	After	% Change
Heart Rate beats per min (bpm)	72	68	- 5.6%
Systolic Blood Pressure mm/Hg	125	120	- 4.0%
Diastolic Blood Pressure mm/Hg	81	75	- 7.4%

None of the individuals included in this table was on blood pressure lowering medication. However, many of my patients on such medications have lowered their blood pressures to the extent that they can also lower their dose of medication or eliminate the need for drugs altogether. I especially encourage those with high blood pressure to monitor their pressures, since that's the only way to really know what it is.

NOTE:
With exercise, many patients lower their blood pressures so they no longer need medication.

The gold standard for determining your aerobic capacity is to measure your oxygen consumption with a gas mask while you exercise on a treadmill or bicycle. Or, you could <u>estimate</u> your oxygen consumption with simpler tests. I'll teach you how to do this with an easy to perform one mile walk test in the companion manual to this book (1).

You could also have your doctor conduct a treadmill test which provides valuable information about your fitness status. For example, Figure 2.4 shows the average exercise heart rates of over 150 participants tested before and after our exercise program. Their heart rates (HR) are plotted on the vertical axis while the time they exercised on the treadmill is indicated on the horizontal line. Every three minutes the work load, that is the grade and speed of the treadmill, was increased at which time their heart rates were measured. The top line shows their average heart rates before they entered the program, and the bottom line shows their results after three months of exercise.

Their heart rates were significantly lower at each stage of the test after the training. Also, you may notice that after the program a greater number of them were able to exercise for a longer time on the treadmill. Indeed, two people ran for 15 minutes . . . a remarkable feat in view of the speed and incline of the treadmill at that stage.

Figure 2.4
IMPROVEMENTS IN HEART RATES
During Treadmill Testing

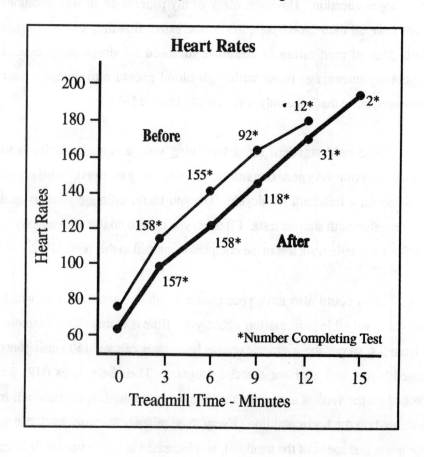

Figure 2.5 shows a similar graph and improvements in the systolic blood pressures of this group in response to fitness training. Their systolic blood pressures are shown on the vertical axis, and the horizontal line indicates the same workload as in the above figure. Notice again, that the average systolic pressure, the pounding force of blood exerted against the wall of all the vessels in your body, can be markedly reduced with only three months of exercise training.

Figure 2.5
IMPROVEMENTS IN SYSTOLIC BLOOD PRESSURES
During Treadmill Testing

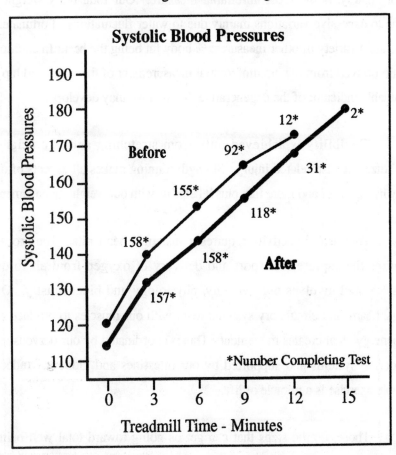

Summary

Physical fitness is an integrated balance of body composition, flexibility, strength and aerobics. You must engage in activities unique to each category in order to achieve total fitness well being. The benefits, however, are well worth the effort and include improvements in both the quantity and quality of your life.

Body composition is commonly measured by body weight which, unfortunately, is the most unreliable measure. Our total body weight is prone to excessive variations mainly due to water fluctuations. Fortunately, there are a variety of other measures; % body fat being the best. In addition, a ratio derived from the circumferential measurement of the waist and hip is a valuable indicator of the degenerative diseases we may develop.

Flexibility is achieved only from stretching and is crucial to minimize exercise related injury. Strength training makes all aspects of our daily living easier and more fun, plus it helps us with our weight management.

True aerobic activity requires a sustained heart rate. The process requires the capture, transport and delivery of oxygen from air to our muscles, and involves our anatomy, physiology and biochemistry. Our lungs, hearts and circulatory systems work with our muscles to produce the "bioenergy" that creates movement. This is coordinated by our nervous and endocrine systems and supported by our intestines and kidneys. Indeed, aerobic exercise is a miracle of life.

Those are the steps that can get us going toward total well being. And, when we make a commitment to these simple principles, we gain the quality of a longer life . . . for the rest of our lives!

Practical Applications

The following is a condensation of the manual, **Total Well Being Through Physical Fitness**, which I am writing as a companion to this book (1). I've included this information here hoping that you will get started with exercise <u>now</u>!

Medical Clearance

To achieve proper medical clearance, go through the screening questionnaire below, Table 2.7. If you answer "yes" to any one of the questions, consult with your physician before doing any exercise.

Table 2.7
SCREENING PRIOR TO BEGINNING EXERCISE*

		YES	NO
1.	Has a doctor ever said you have high blood pressure or a heart condition?		
2.	Has a doctor ever recommended medication for your blood pressure or for a heart condition?		
3.	Have you ever felt forceful or rapid beats in your heart?		
4.	Has a doctor ever said you have a heart murmur?		
5.	Have you ever had chest pain brought on by physical exertion?		
6.	Have you ever had unaccustomed shortness of breath at rest, or with mild exertion?		
7.	Have you ever had difficulty sleeping or lying down due to shortness of breath?		
8.	Have you ever lost consciousness or fallen over as a result of dizziness?		
9.	Have you ever had recurrent swelling in your ankles?		
10.	Have you ever had recurrent pain in your legs with physical exertion?		

11. Do you have a bone or joint problem that could be aggravated by physical activity?

12. Are you pregnant?

13. Are you aware, through your own experience or a doctor's advice, of any other physical reason against your exercising without medical supervision?

*Adapted from: Shephard, R.J. et al. *The Canadian Home Fitness Test.* SportsMed. 1991; 11:358-366 and American College of Sports Medicine. **Guidelines for Exercise Testing and Prescription.** Lea & Febiger, Philadelphia, PA. 1991, 4th ed.

Stretching

NOTE:
I cannot emphasize enough the importance of stretching both before and after exercise to prevent musculoskeletal injury.

I cannot emphasize enough the importance of stretching both before and after exercise to prevent musculoskeletal injury. That is why I've designed and choreographed the 16 stretches below that work your entire body. When you do them properly, it will insure your maximum benefit and safety.

Your Stretching Routine

Although there is some controversy regarding when you should stretch, based upon my own personal and professional experience, I recommend stretching in two phases: 1) Pre-exercise, focused muscle stretch, and 2) Post-exercise, total body stretch. To minimize injury during your pre-exercise stretch, I suggest that you do what I practice and recommend to my patients . . . warm up first.

Pre-Exercise Stretch

The pre-exercise stretch consists of a brief warm-up followed by stretching the major muscle groups you will be using in your exercise routine.

Warm-Up

Warm up for three to five minutes prior to stretching. This increases your heart rate and gets your circulation going so blood can warm up your muscles and prepare your body to stretch. If I'm at the Institute, I either ride a stationary bike, walk on a treadmill or do light exercises on some other apparatus. If I'm outside, I do some easy walking or very light jogging in place. A few abdominal curls and pushups also gets the circulatory system going. After this gentle warm up, I do the focus muscle stretches.

Focus Muscle Stretch

After warming up, concentrate on stretching those muscles you will incorporate in your upcoming exercise. For example, if you plan to do weight training, focus on those muscles which will be utilized during your lifting. For aerobics, such as walk/jog, you'll want to stretch your legs and lower back. After all, what muscles are in constant contraction in those of us who sit in an office all day . . . hamstrings, buttocks and lower back muscles. Stretch slowly - never bounce - and hold the stretch for 10 - 20 seconds.

NOTE:
. . . Stretch slowly - never bounce . . . and hold the stretch for 10-20 seconds.

Post-Exercise Stretching

After exercising, you have probably noticed that your flexibility is markedly increased. Take advantage of warm muscles to maintain and further increase your flexibility by going through your entire stretching routine. This post-stretch will definitely reduce your chances of muscle soreness the next time out.

Proper Body Alignment and Breathing

NOTE:
. . . listen to your body as you move.

As you stretch, pay special attention to your body alignment and breathing. Keep your back straight, and move with a slow controlled motion. Pay attention to your breathing and listen to your body as you move. This will help develop your body-mind connection; a pathway toward total well being.

Active Stretching

I call this system "Active Stretching." It is a combination of regular stretching and Yoga that enables you to concentrate on your body and, at the same time, heighten the awareness of your mind. It's a tool that uses your body as a pathway to the integration and balance you need to feel totally well.

Exercises

1. **SHOULDER SHRUGS** (Photograph 2.1).

    - Stand with your feet hip width apart and arms comfortably by your sides (the standing position).
    - Inhale.
    - Exhale as you bring your shoulders up to your ears (Photograph 2.1).
    - Inhale as you slowly relax your shoulders to a resting position.
    - Repeat 3 - 5 times.

Photograph 2.1

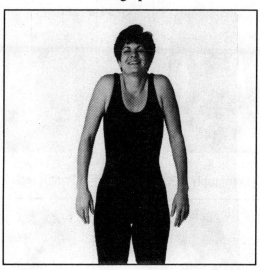

2. **NECK STRETCH** (Photographs 2.2A, 2.2B, 2.2C, and 2.2D).

    - In the standing position, inhale.
    - Exhale as you slowly drop your right ear toward your right shoulder (Photograph 2.2A).
    - Inhale as you bring your head up to the resting position.

- Exhale as you slowly drop your left ear toward your left shoulder (Photograph 2.2B).

- Inhale as you bring your head up to the resting position.

- Exhale as you slowly drop your chin toward your chest (Photograph 2.2C).

- Inhale as you bring your head up to the resting position.

- Exhale as you slowly drop your head backward (Photograph 2.2D).

- Inhale as you bring your head up to the resting position.

- Repeat the sequence 3 - 5 times.

NOTE:
Use slow controlled movements.

Photograph 2.2A

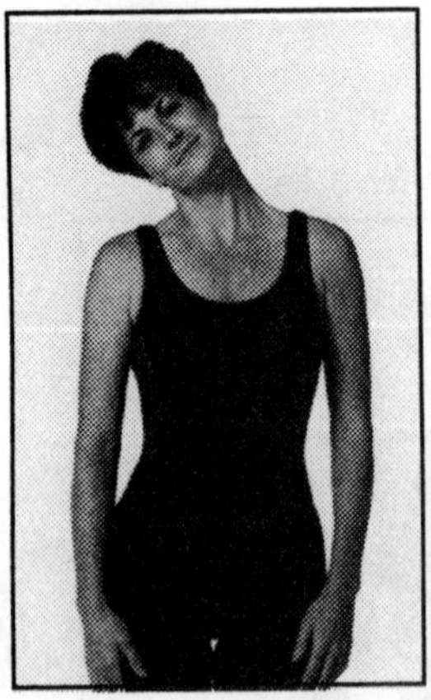

Photograph 2.2B

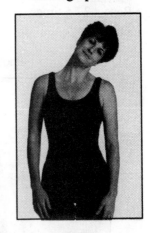

Photograph 2.2C

Photograph 2.2D

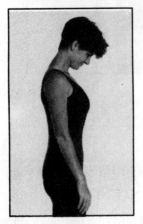

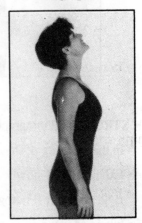

Use slow controlled movements. Do not bend your head too far **back.** Notice the breathing pattern and feel your body as you stretch.

3. UPPER EXTREMITIES - FRONT (Photograph 2.3).

- In the standing position, raise your right arm up in front of you to shoulder height.
- Bend at your elbow, moving your forearm in toward chest.
- Reach your left hand under and behind your right elbow.
- Inhale.
- Exhale as you draw your right arm across your chest applying pressure with your left hand (Photograph 2.3).
- Breathe as you release.

Photograph 2.3

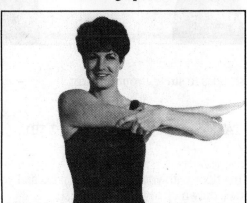

- Reverse sides to stretch your left arm.

4. UPPER EXTREMITIES - OVERHEAD (Photographs 2.4A and 2.4B).

- From the standing position, raise your right arm straight up.
- Bend at your elbow and slowly drop your hand back between your shoulder blades.

- Bring your left hand up and grasp your right elbow (Photographs 2.4A and 2.4B).

- Inhale.

- Exhale as you draw your right elbow toward the mid-line of your back (Photographs 2.4A and 2.4B).

- Breathe as you release.

Photograph 2.4A   Photograph 2.4B

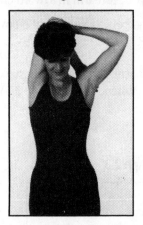   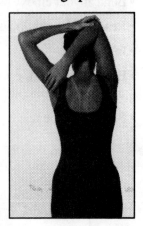

- Reverse sides to stretch your left arm.

5. SPINAL ROTATION (Photographs 2.5A and 2.5B).

- Sit on the floor with your left leg extended and your right knee drawn up toward your chest.

- Cross your right leg over your left leg and plant your right foot on the floor, just outside your left knee.

- Place your right hand on the floor behind you.

- Cross your left elbow in front of and to the outside of your right knee.

- Inhale.

- Exhale as you rotate your upper body toward the right, looking over your right shoulder (Photographs 2.5A).

- Breathe as you release.

Photograph 2.5A

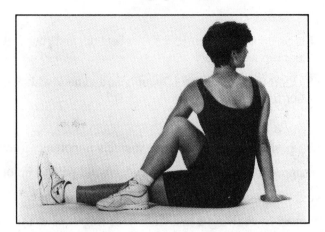

NOTE:
This is one exercise where it's particularly beneficial to listen to your body.

• Reverse sides to stretch your right side (Photograph 2.5B).

Photograph 2.5B

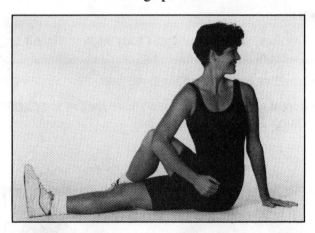

This is one exercise where it's particularly beneficial to listen to your body. Spinal rotation involves a lot of stretching and compressing which stimulates the nerve endings from your spine, and consequently, thousands of nerve endings throughout your body. All of the cells that are stimulated, in turn, send messages back to your brain. This dynamic circuit of excitation and feedback going on in your nervous system gives you a marvelous opportunity to tap into the mind - body connection, that is, if you allow yourself to "listen."

6. ABDOMINAL CURLS - STRAIGHT (Photograph 2.6).

- Lie on your back with your knees bent up, and your feet on the floor hip width apart.
- Support the bottom part of your head and neck with your fingertips.

The position of your hands is extremely important. They are placed strictly to support the weight of your head. Avoid pulling up on your head which would cause your neck to flex, or bend forward. Visualize the triangle formed by drawing a line from your fingertips at the base of your head over to your elbows, and then down your arms to your shoulders. As you curl, raise that triangle up as a unit.

- Inhale.
- Exhale as you lift your upper body a few inches off the floor (Photograph 2.6).
- Inhale as you release back to the floor.
- Repeat as many times as you can so long as you <u>maintain</u> <u>proper</u> <u>form</u>.

NOTE:
The position of your hands is extremely important. They are placed strictly to support the weight of your head.

Photograph 2.6

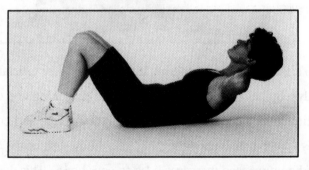

The most important movement in this exercise is to raise your head, neck, shoulders and arms in unison. The longer and slower the exhalation, the deeper the action in the abdominal muscles. As you exhale and lift up, feel the contraction in your lower abdomen and feel the small of your back move toward the floor.

Also, remember to breathe properly. Breathing is extremely important, since this is a strengthening maneuver as much as a stretch. Breathe out as you come up to avoid increasing your blood pressure.

NOTE:
Breathe out as you come up to avoid increasing your blood pressure.

7. PELVIC TILTS (Photograph 2.7).

• Begin on your back as in the abdominal curls.

• Place your arms alongside your body with your hands on your abdomen.

• Inhale.

• Exhale as you contract your lower abdominal muscles, forcing the small of your back toward the floor and raising the lower part of your pelvis up (Photograph 2.7).

• Inhale as you release.

• Repeat as many times as you did the abdominal curls.

Photograph 2.7

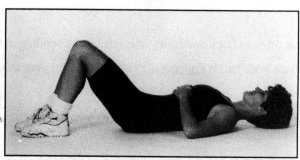

8. ABDOMINAL CURLS - TRANSVERSE (Photograph 2.8).

- Begin on your back, as you did with the abdominal curls.

- Inhale.

- Exhale as you raise your right shoulder and arm tracking your right side to the upper outside of your left knee (Photograph 2.8).

- Inhale as you relax back to the floor.

- Repeat these curls as many times as you can, so long as you maintain proper form.

Photograph 2.8

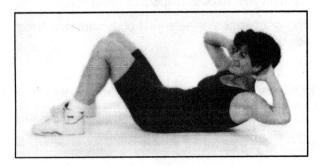

- Reverse sides to work the left transverse abdominal muscles .

9. KNEE TO CHEST (Photographs 2.9A and 2.9B).

- Lie on your back and raise your left leg up bending at the knee.

- Place your hands underneath your leg behind your thigh.

- Inhale.

- Exhale as you bring your left knee to your chest (Photograph 2.9A).

- Inhale as you release your foot back to the floor.

Photograph 2.9A

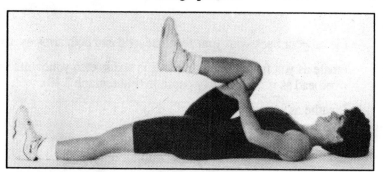

Notice that your hands are under your leg rather than wrapped around on top. This prevents you from forcing your knee into severe flexion. The way to protect your joints is to avoid forcing them into extreme angles. You want to always maintain what we call "soft joints."

• Reverse sides to work your right leg.

• Now, bring both legs up to your chest and fold your arms behind both legs.

• Inhale.

• Press both knees to your chest (Photograph 2.9B).

• Breathe as you release.

Photograph 2.9B

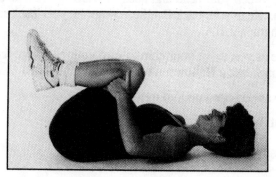

10. TALL EXTENSION (Photograph 2.10).

- Lie on your back with your feet extended and both arms overhead.
- Inhale as you further extend your legs and stretch your arms as far overhead as is comfortably possible (Photograph 2.10).
- Breathe as you release.

Photograph 2.10

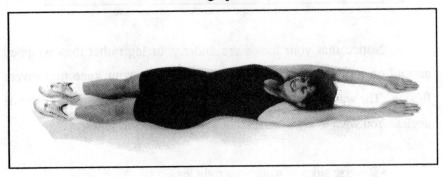

11. DOG AND CAT (Photographs 2.11A and 2.11B).

Using your hands and arms for support, slowly roll over from your resting position on the floor to your hands and knees in what is called the table, or dog position.

- Gently sweep your head and neck forward as you take in a deep breath. Keep your back flat, i.e., do not let your back sag (Photograph 2.11A).
- Exhale as you move your chin toward your chest and arch your back like a Halloween cat (Photograph 2.11B).
- Inhale as you open up into the dog position.
- Repeat 3 - 5 times.

Photograph 2.11A

Photograph 2.11B

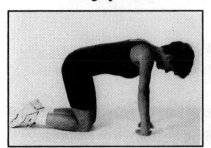
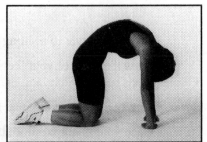

12. DOG AND CAT VARIATION (Photographs 2.12A and 21.2B).

- Inhale as you draw your chest up and out and, this time, extend your right leg straight back keeping your back flat (Photograph 2.12A).

- Exhale and compress by bringing your chin toward your chest and bending your right knee in toward your forehead (Photograph 2.12B).

- Inhale back into the straight-legged dog position.

- Then exhale into the cat with an arched back.

- Alternate legs so that the left leg is extended out with inhalation, and then drawn in toward your forehead with exhalation.

- Repeat the sequence 3 - 5 times.

Photograph 2.12A

Photograph 2.12B

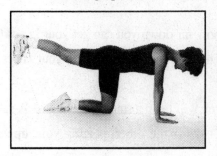
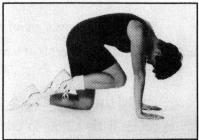

13. ADDUCTOR (GROIN) STRETCH (Photograph 2.13).

- Slowly roll over to a sitting position.
- Draw the soles of your feet toward each other and place your hands behind you.
- Slowly lift yourself up and gently slide forward toward your feet.
- Place your hands comfortably in front of you on your feet.
- Inhale.
- Exhale and slowly push your feet together and extend from your groin out toward your knees (Photograph 2.13).
- Inhale as you release.

Photograph 2.13

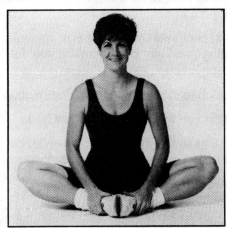

This is not a movement of how far down you can get your knees to the floor. Think of it in terms of lengthening from your groin to your knees.

For the last three stretches, you will be in a standing position. A safe way to get up is by rolling to one side or the other, placing your upper, outside foot on the floor. For example, if you roll toward your left side, place your right foot on the floor and support your weight with your left hand. Balance yourself with your right hand on your right knee (Photograph 2.S1).

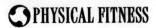

Come to a kneeling position on your left knee and place both of your hands on your right knee for support (Photograph 2.S2).

Then, bring your other foot up onto the floor to a standing position.

Photograph 2.S1

Photograph 2.S2

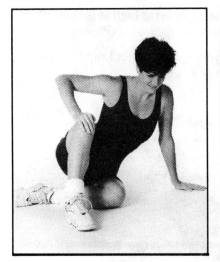

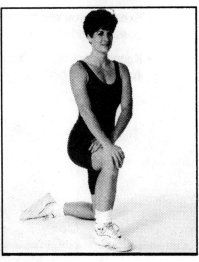

14. HAMSTRINGS (Photograph 2.14).

- Step forward with your left foot.

- Keep your right knee slightly bent and place your hands just above your knee for support and balance.

- Inhale.

- Exhale as you reach your left toes up as high as is comfortably possible and move your buttocks backward (Photograph 2.14).

- Keep the entire length of your spine straight from your lower back to your neck. Inhale as you release.

Photograph 2.14

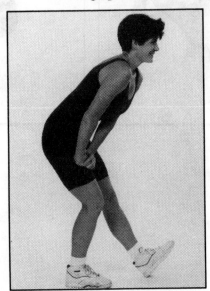

- Reverse sides to stretch your right hamstring.

15. QUADRICEPS (Photograph 2.15).

- Support yourself with your left hand on a chair or wall.

- Clasp your right heel with your right hand.

- Inhale.

- Exhale as you move your bent right leg backward and your
  right hip forward (Photograph 2.15).

Photograph 2.15

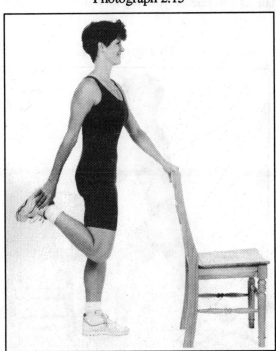

Notice that you should not place your hand under your foot. That way you do not pull up on your foot, which could put too much flexion and strain on your knee. Remember, you want to maintain "soft joints." Again, the action here is to move your leg backward while pushing the right side of your pelvis forward.

- Reverse sides to stretch your left quadriceps.

16. GASTROCNEMIUS (CALF MUSCLE) and ACHILLES TENDON
(Photograph 2.16).

• Support yourself with your hands on a chair or wall.

• Step back as far as is comfortable onto the ball of your right foot.

• Inhale.

• Exhale and slowly press your right heel to the floor bringing the heel of your right foot all the way down to the floor (Photograph 2.16).

• Inhale as you release your leg forward.

Photograph 2.16

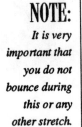

NOTE:
It is very important that you do not bounce during this or any other stretch.

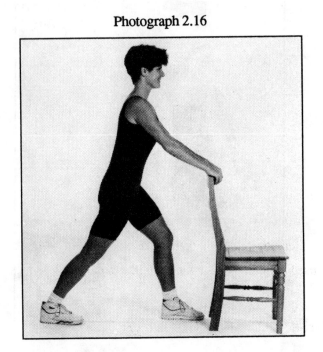

• Reverse sides to stretch your left calf muscle.

It is very important that you do not bounce during this or any other stretch. Bouncing during this stretch could injure your Achilles tendon. In fact, all stretches should be done slowly, without bouncing, feeling an active deep stretch without pain.

Strengthening

Strength training balances your body alignment, creates symmetry and flexibility and enhances your ability to perform aerobic activities. It enables you to perform daily tasks with increased ease, agility and vigor. More importantly, you will look and feel better than you've ever looked or felt before.

Like all exercises, strength training must be done <u>properly</u> in order to be safe. Before you begin the exercises in this chapter, read the next few paragraphs carefully so that you can apply these principles as you learn each of the exercises.

NOTE:
Like all exercises, strength training must be done <u>properly</u> in order to be safe.

Equipment

Since free weights are relatively inexpensive and easy to use, they are best suited for your home exercise. I discourage the use of barbells unless you work out with someone who can act as a spotter. Single free weights, or dumbbells, can be just as effective and are much safer, which is why I've used them in creating the exercises in this section.

Dumbbells

You can choose from two kinds of dumbbells. The first kind is premolded with a fixed weight. These are the easiest to use, but you will need several pairs with different weights to accommodate the various lifts in your routine. The second kind is a short bar with detachable weights which offer more flexibility in that you can change weights as needed. It is, however, inconvenient to interrupt your routine to make that adjustment.

The most common adjustable weight dumbbells are those found in a department store. They usually come in a set with enough weights to accommodate the beginner. The weights are secured with a bolted collar which is safe if properly tightened. However, the bar is usually 13 inches long which may not give you enough clearance as you move the dumbbell along side of the chair or bench you use for support.

More expensive, professional type dumbbells can be purchased with a 10 inch bar. However, these weights are attached with end screws that are not easily removed. Moreover, the bar requires two or more weight plates at each end, so you need a greater variety of plates to create the weight required for different exercises.

You will need to decide what type of dumbbells you should obtain. Initially, you will probably want a combination of both fixed and variable weights.

For example, you will probably need 5-25 pounds per dumbbell. I suggest one pair of fixed weights at 8 pounds and another at 15 pounds. In addition, I recommend one pair of variable weights up to 25 pounds. These three different sets of dumbbells will allow you to move smoothly through your exercise routine.

The Chair

For support, I recommend you use a solidly built, straight back chair. Sitting upright and back into the chair gives you protection against lower back injury, which is a common problem associated with poor form when weight-lifting. If possible, use a narrow chair, approximately 15 inches wide, for clearance of movement on both sides.

Principles of Proper Strength Training

Applying proper principles while strength training is mandatory in order to insure your safety. This includes proper form with attention to body alignment, the right breathing pattern with exhalation during the exertion phase and slow, easy movements throughout the exercises.

Form

Correct form is crucial for safe strength training, and you can maintain proper form by paying attention to proper body alignment. Indeed, misalignment or awkward body position is the major cause of musculoskeletal injury during weight lifting. A classic example is when people strain during an overhead lift and arch their backs to get that last little push completely up. Your goal should be to improve your overall muscular strength. Lifting heavier and heavier weights simply to prove you can beat your last effort or the effort of someone else is asking for trouble.

These exercises are designed to work both sides of your body together, symmetrically. This principle helps you maintain proper body alignment. In addition, there is an alternating pattern of push/pull similar to your stretching exercises. This approach forces you to pay attention to proper form and to concentrate on separate muscle groups as well as your whole body working as a system. Then, as you add proper breathing to the exercises, as in your stretching routines, you have an opportunity to tune into the messages from your body.

NOTE:
. . . misalignment or awkward body position is the major cause of musculoskeletal injury during weight lifting.

Breathing

The most important component of strength training, often the most overlooked or incorrectly done, is proper breathing. To breathe correctly, you must exhale during exertion and inhale with recovery. Breathing in the opposite way is extremely harmful, because you can dangerously increase your blood pressure.

Slow, Easy, Controlled Movements

Use slow, easy, controlled movements! A good way to do this is to follow the two to four ratio. Slowly count to two during contraction and to four during the relaxation phase. Avoid the temptation of swinging the weights, especially during the release phase of the lift. This can cause rapid, jerky movements ... the kind that lead to muscle tears.

Exercise Progression

It's important to begin the strengthening exercises with light weights and gradually increase weights, repetitions (reps) and sets. Reps are consecutive exertions for each exercise, for example 10-12 lifts per exercise.

Guidelines for a strength training progression are given in Table 2.8. Begin with 1-5 pounds the first week and concentrate on learning proper technique. For the next few weeks use enough weight to reach exhaustion at the end of 10-12 reps for each exercise. If you feel comfortable after approximately four weeks, do two sets for each exercise. Allow two to three minutes between sets. Since you will be doing up to as many as 24

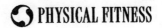

repetitions, you will need to decrease the weight so that you can maintain proper form during the last few repetitions. As you gain more experience, you will be able to move up to three sets per exercise. Again, readjust the weights so that you exhaust yourself but keep proper form during your last repetitions. Remember, to exercise <u>properly</u> is to exercise <u>safely</u>!

NOTE:
. . . to exercise properly is to exercise safely!

Table 2.8
STRENGTH TRAINING PROGRESSION

Week	Weight	Reps	Sets per Exercise	Notes
1	1 - 5 lbs	10 - 12	1	To learn proper technique
2-4	To exhaustion	10 - 12	1	Maintain proper form at last rep
4-8	To exhaustion	10 - 12	2	Decrease weights as you increase sets
>8	To exhaustion	10 - 12	3	Decrease weights as you increase sets

Exercises

1. HEEL RAISES (Photograph 2.17).

   Muscles: Gastrocnemius (Calf Muscle).

   - Hold a dumbbell in your right hand, with your palm facing in.
   - Support yourself with your left hand on a chair or against the wall.
   - Keep your body erect and your head up.
   - Place your weight on your right leg by lifting your left foot up and resting it on the back of your right heel.
   - Inhale.
   - Exhale as you lift your weight up on the ball of your right foot and hold momentarily (Photograph 2.17).
   - Inhale as you relax your foot back to the floor.

Photograph 2.17

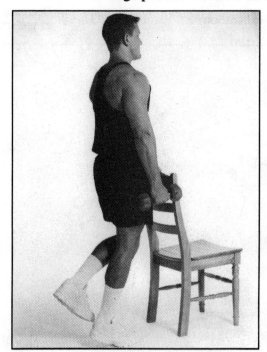

   - Reverse sides to exercise your left calf muscle.

2. WALL SQUAT (Photograph 2.18).

   Muscles: Quadriceps, along the front of your thighs.

   - Hold dumbbells in both hands with your arms hanging along your sides.
   - Keep your palms in and stand with your back supported against a wall.
   - Place your feet 12 to 18 inches from the wall and hip width apart with your toes pointed forward.
   - Inhale as you slowly lower your body.
   - Come to a sitting position, which is just short of creating a right angle between your back and thighs (Photograph 2.18).
   - Never allow your knees to move forward of your feet.
   - Exhale as you move back up into the standing position.

Photograph 2.18

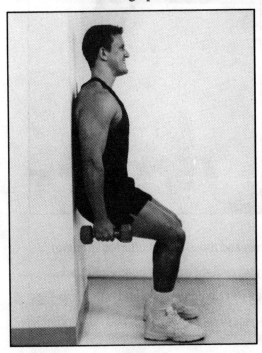

3. PUSH UPS (Photographs 2.19A, 2.19B and 2.19C).
   Muscles: Pectorals, along your upper front chest; Arms, both biceps and triceps; Abdominals.

   Beginners:

   • Stand next to the wall at arms length.

   • Support yourself against the wall with your arms at shoulder width.

   • Inhale and move closer to the wall.

   • Exhale and slowly push yourself away from the wall (Photograph 2.19A).

Photograph 2.19A

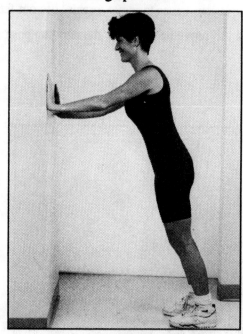

Most women and those with moderate strength:

   • Support your weight on your hands and knees.

   • Raise your feet up behind you and cross your legs.

   • Inhale as you slowly lower your body to a point just above the floor.

   • Exhale as you push up with your arms (Photograph 2.19B).

Photograph 2.19B

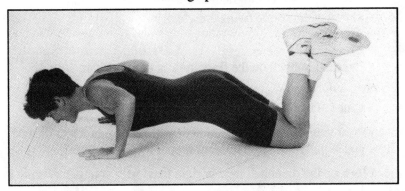

Advanced:

• Support your weight on your hands and toes.

• Keep your hands shoulder width apart.

• Inhale as you slowly move downward.

• Exhale as you slowly push up (Photograph 2.19C).

NOTE:
Exhale as you slowly push up.

Photograph 2.19C

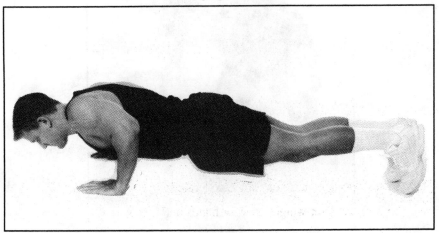

4. ONE SIDED RAISE (Photograph 2.20).
   Muscles: Latasimus dorsi (wing muscles).

- Place a dumbbell on the floor in front of your chair.

- Face the side of your chair and support yourself with your left hand.

- Plant your feet firmly on the floor with your right leg to the rear and slightly out for maximum support.

- Pick up the dumbbell in your right hand with your palm facing in.

- Keep the weight directly under your shoulder.

- Inhale.

- Exhale as you pull the weight straight up to your side keeping your arm close to your body (Photograph 2.20).

- Inhale as you lower the weight back to a resting position.

Photograph 2.20

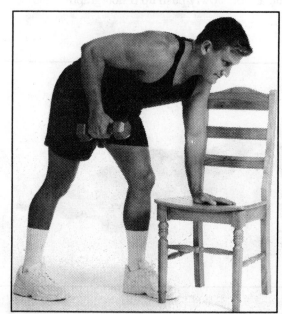

- Reverse positions to work your wing muscles on the left side.

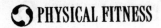

5. PECTORAL FLYS (Photograph 2.21).

Muscles: Pectorals, along the front of your chest.

- Lie down with your upper back and head on two pillows to give your arms room to stretch downward without hitting the floor.

- Bring your feet up and rest them on the floor hip width apart.

- Hold the dumbbells in both hands with your palms up.

- Inhale.

- Exhale and slowly raise the weights up over your chest (Photograph 2.21).

- Inhale as you slowly guide your hands back to a point just above the floor.

Photograph 2.21

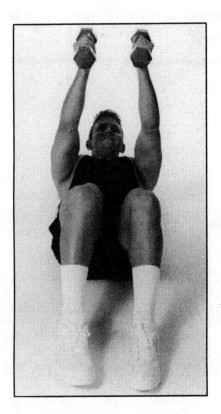

6. ABDOMINAL CURLS - STRAIGHT.

Muscles: Longitudinal and transverse abdominal and pelvic girdle.

- Review the abdominal curls straight, page 72.

7. PELVIC TILTS.

Muscles: Abdominal and lower back muscles.

- Review the pelvic tilts, page 73.

8. ABDOMINAL CURLS - TRANSVERSE.

Muscles: Transverse abdominals, muscles on the sides of your abdomen.

- Review the abdominal curls transverse, page 74.

9. LATERAL RAISES (Photograph 2.22).

Muscles: Deltoids, along the top of your shoulders.

- Sit back in the chair to support your back.

- Plant your feet firmly on the floor.

- Hold the dumbbells in both hands with your palms facing in and arms straight down at your sides.

- Inhale.

- Exhale as you slowly raise the dumbbells to a point even with your shoulders (Photograph 2.22).

- Inhale as you slowly return to the starting position.

Photograph 2.22

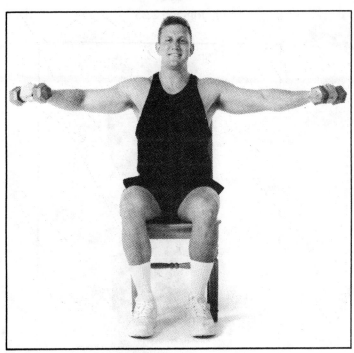

10. OVERHEAD PRESS (Photograph 2.23).

Muscles: Deltoids and trapezius, posterior neck muscles.

• Sit back in the chair to support your back.

• Plant your feet firmly on the floor.

• Lift the dumbbells to your shoulders with your palms
  facing forward.

• Inhale.

• Exhale and press the dumbbells overhead, bringing the weights
  close together at the top (Photograph 2.23).

• Inhale as you lower the dumbbells back to the level of your
  shoulders.

Photograph 2.23

NOTE:
*. . . avoid the
natural tendency
of arching your
lower back.*

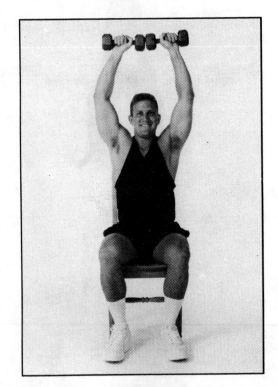

Keep your arms in the same lateral plane with your body and avoid
the natural tendency of arching your lower back.

11. SHOULDER SHRUGS (Photograph 2.24).

Muscles: Deltoids, trapezius, and shoulder girdle muscles.

- Stand with your feet hip width apart.
- Hold dumbbells in both hands along your sides with your palms facing in.
- Inhale.
- Exhale as you slowly raise your shoulders up (Photograph 2.24).
- Hesitate at the top and feel the squeeze in your muscles.
- Inhale as you slowly lower the weights back to the resting position.

Photograph 2.24

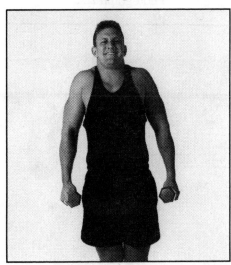

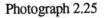

12. BICEPS CURL (Photograph 2.25).

Muscles: Biceps, along the front of your upper arm.

- Sit back in the chair to support your back.
- Plant your feet firmly on the floor.
- Hold the dumbbells at arm's length, palms facing inward.
- Inhale.
- Exhale and curl both weights up, rotating your arms so that your palms face toward the rear at the top of the lift (Photo 2.25).
- Inhale as you return to the resting position.

Photograph 2.25

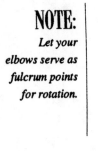

NOTE:
Let your elbows serve as fulcrum points for rotation.

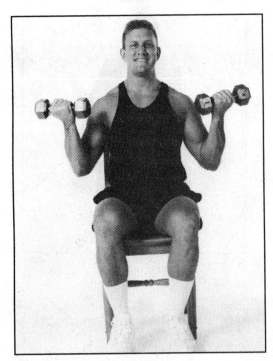

To isolate the movement in the biceps, keep your elbows pinned at the same point along your sides throughout the rotation up. Let your elbows serve as fulcrum points for rotation.

13. TRICEPS CURL (Photograph 2.26).

Muscles: Triceps, along the back of your upper arm.

- Place a dumbbell on the floor in front of your chair.

- Face the side of your chair and support yourself with your left hand.

- Plant your feet firmly on the floor with your right leg to the rear and slightly out for maximum support.

- Lift the dumbbell up with your right hand, palm facing in, so that your elbow is above your shoulder.

- Inhale.

- Exhale as you press the weight backward and up, keeping your elbow pinned above your side to isolate the action in your triceps. (Photograph 2.26).

- Inhale as you return the weight down below your elbow.

Photograph 2.26

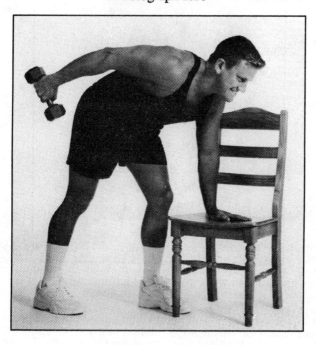

- Reverse sides to work your left triceps muscle.

14. WRIST CURLS (Photograph 2.27).

Muscles: Forearm, along the underside of your lower arm.

- Sit in your chair and hold a dumbbell in your right hand palm facing up.
- Place the back of your forearm on your right thigh with your hand and weight hanging over the end of your knee.
- Give your forearm support with your left hand.
- Inhale.
- Exhale and slowly curl the dumbbell up as high as is comfortably possible (Photograph 2.27).
  - Inhale back to the beginning position.

Photograph 2.27

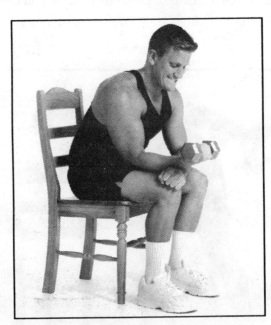

- Reverse sides to work your left forearm muscles.

These exercises that strengthen your wrists and forearms are particularly valuable for tennis players and golfers.

Aerobics

As I have discussed, aerobic exercise is one of the best activities you can do since it improves so many functions in your body. However, any aerobic activity must be done properly to avoid minor injuries, as well as potentially fatal medical problems.

During aerobics, your body converts fat into energy, which sustains exercises such as walking, swimming, bicycling, stepping, jogging and other continuous activities. During these activities, energy is provided by the breakdown of fats in the presence of oxygen. The key to gaining benefits from aerobic exercise is the length of time you <u>sustain</u> the exercise.

NOTE:
The key to gaining benefits from aerobic exercise is the length of time you <u>sustain</u> the exercise.

Your Aerobic Session

To be safe and minimize injury, think of an aerobic session as one which includes a sequence of activities, including the following steps:

Step 1.	Warm-Up	2 - 5 minutes
Step 2.	Pre-Exercise Stretch	5 - 10 minutes
Step 3.	Aerobics Phase	25 - 30 minutes
Step 4.	Cool-Down	3 - 5 minutes
Step 5.	Post-Exercise Stretch	10 - 20 minutes

Step 1. Warm-Up.

This involves light aerobic activity to get your circulation going and warm up your muscles in preparation for stretching.

Step 2. Pre-Exercise Stretch.

Focus your stretch on those muscles that you will mainly rely upon in your aerobic activity. Generally, they include the quadriceps, hamstrings, and calf muscles.

Step 3. Aerobic Phase.

Discussed later in this chapter.

Step 4. Cool-Down.

NOTE:
Cool-down will help reduce soreness the next time out.

As important as it is to "start your engine," it is equally important to cool down. Your cardiovascular system is revved up as you work in your training heart zone. If you were to stop suddenly, blood would pool in your extremities causing low blood pressure and light headedness. Furthermore, you need a gradual slowing in order to wash out the lactic acid and other toxic wastes that have built up during exercise. This will help reduce soreness the next time out. Lastly, if you stop your physical activity abruptly, there is a sudden rebound of adrenaline. Excessive adrenaline may produce erratic heart rhythms which could lead to serious medical problems.

To cool down, reverse the warm-up activities that you did or simply taper down your aerobic exercise. Monitor your heart rate and note how fast you return to your resting heart rate. In fact, the best indicator of your fitness level is how fast you recover after exercise.

Step 5. Post-Exercise Stretch.

Go through your total body stretches when your muscles and tendons are thoroughly warmed up and most capable of being fully stretched.

Intensity

Regardless of the activity, the intensity with which you exercise is the most critical factor relating to your safety. This includes minor injuries as well as serious medical problems, even fatalities. In Chapter 2, I discussed the positive association between strenuous activity and heart attacks in sedentary people. Intensity is the component of exercise that puts these people at risk.

NOTE:
... intensity ... is the most critical factor relating to your safety.

Exercise science has designed an accurate way to monitor your exercise intensity so that you can exercise in a safe aerobic zone by monitoring your heart rate. We call this your training heart rate (THR).

The most profound advice I can give you on how to exercise safely is to know <u>your</u> area of discomfort and <u>your</u> region of pain. Avoid moving from discomfort into pain. If you do, move out of pain by stopping your activity and don't do it again!

You will need to learn how to take your heart rate, or pulse, in applying these principles. So, follow the directions below.

Radial Pulse

Refer to Photo 2.28 to see how to take your radial pulse. Allow your left hand to relax with your palm up. With the pads of your right index and middle fingers, follow a point from the base of your left thumb up about one inch. Feel for your pulse. It can be felt just on the outside of the stringy tendons that are in the middle part of your wrist. Many people find that by turning their watches to the underside of their wrists, it is easier to keep time.

Photograph 2.28

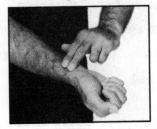

Carotid Pulse

Now, practice feeling for the carotid pulse in your neck. Using your index and middle fingers, find your voice box and then move about an eighth of an inch to the outside, Photograph 2.29. Do not press too hard and palpate only one side at a time.

Photograph 2.29

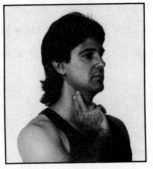

Resting Heart Rate

To practice monitoring your pulse, take your resting heart rate. Palpate either your radial or carotid pulse while using a time piece. At the mark, begin to count each pulsation up to one minute. This gives you your resting heart rate in beats per minute.

The 15 Second Count

Now, imagine that you are exercising, and your heart rate is accelerated. If you stop and measure your pulse for a full minute, your heart rate would slow down as you recovered from the activity. Therefore, you would not really know what your heart rate was during your exercise. However, you can overcome this error by immediately doing a 15 second count. Get your timing device ready, monitor your pulse and at the mark, begin by counting each pulsation for 15 seconds. Multiply that number by four to obtain your heart rate in beats per minute. You could also refer to Table 2.9 which makes the conversion for you.

Table 2.9
CONVERSION OF HEART RATE (HR)
From beats per minute to beats per 15 seconds. Use during exercise.

HR Minutes	HR 15 Seconds	HR Minutes	HR 15 Seconds
100	25	140	35
102	26	142	36
104	26	144	36
106	27	146	37
108	27	148	37
110	28	150	38
112	28	152	38
114	29	154	39
116	29	156	39
118	30	158	40
120	30	160	40
122	31	162	41
124	31	164	41
126	32	166	42
128	32	168	42
130	33	170	43
132	33	172	43
134	34	174	44
136	34	176	44
138	35	178	45
140	35	180	45

Estimating Your Fitness Category

You will also need to estimate your fitness category before you calculate your THR and later create your own exercise prescription. Estimate your category by matching your level of fitness with the categories below, Table 2.10.

Table 2.10

ESTIMATING YOUR FITNESS CATEGORY

Category	Level of Fitness
Basic	Beginner to exercise.
Maintenance	Been exercising at a mild to moderate level for some time.
Experienced	Been exercising regularly at a moderate to advanced level.

Calculating Your Training Heart Rate in Three Easy Steps

Go through these steps to see how simple it is to determine a training heart rate. Then, fill in Table 2.11 to determine your THR.

STEP ONE:

Determine your maximum heart rate (max HR) by subtracting your age from 220. For example, if you are 50 years old, 220 minus 50 gives you an estimated max HR of 170 beats per minute.

STEP TWO:

Determine your THR by multiplying your max HR by 60 to 85% depending upon your fitness category. Let's assume you are in the Basic category. Use a fitness factor of 60%. Sixty percent times 170 gives you a training heart rate of 102 beats per one minute.

STEP THREE:

Remember that when you are working out, you only need to take your pulse for 15 seconds. The next calculation you must make is to divide the beats per one minute, in this case 102, by four. This gives you your training heart rate in beats per 15 seconds. In this example, the number is 26. Therefore, if you were working out aerobically, your heart rate should be 26 beats in 15 seconds.

Table 2.11
CALCULATE YOUR TRAINING HEART RATE

Steps		Your THR
Description	Formula	Your Calculation
Max HR	(220- AGE)	
THR per min	(Max HR x %) 60% Basic 70% Maintenance 85% Experienced	
THR per 15 sec	(THR ÷ 4)	

NOTE:
... never exceed your training heart rate!

When you first begin exercising and are not yet sensitive to the physical clues from your body, it's imperative that you periodically pause during your workout, walk in place, and measure your 15 second pulse. Then, compare this to your calculated training heart rate. If you are below your THR, that's O.K. It will take you just a little longer to achieve your desired results. The important point is to never exceed your training heart rate!

Listen to Your Body

Over time, listening to your body as you stretch, strengthen and exercise aerobically will make you sensitive to an infinite number of signals and clues about how you feel. As you progress toward total well being, your understanding of your body will become increasingly heightened. You will sense how you feel at the moment by the degree of tension in your jaw . . . the strength and tone in specific muscle groups . . . your lung capacity and heart rate . . . how energized you are.

My FIT Prescription

I want to introduce you to the concept of <u>My</u> <u>FIT</u> <u>P</u>rescription which you can use to create your own prescription for aerobic exercise. In fact, you can apply these principles to stretching and strengthening which is described more fully in the manual. Refer to Table 2.12, page 113, as you learn how this prescription works.

NOTE:
You can apply the principles of <u>My</u> <u>FIT</u> <u>P</u>rescription to aerobics, stretching and strengthening.

The components of <u>My</u> <u>FIT</u> <u>P</u>rescription are:

<u>M</u>odality	- Type of exercise.
<u>F</u>requency	- Number of times you exercise per week.
<u>I</u>ntensity	- Level at which you exercise.
<u>T</u>ime	- Duration of each exercise.
<u>P</u>rogression	- Advancement of your exercise.

Modality

Modality refers to the type of activity that you do. Notice that as you move from the Basic to the Experienced category, the types of activity become more strenuous because they progressively involve more weight-bearing activities. In weight-bearing activities, you use a larger muscle mass and, therefore, burn more calories. For example, walking involves keeping a foot in <u>contact</u> with the ground at all times. Contrast this with jogging where you <u>lift</u> your body off the ground. This is the reason there is such a big jump in caloric expenditure between walking and jogging. You will expend approximately the same number of calories whether you walk or jog any given distance; it just takes less time if you move faster.

Notice that I recommend only walking in the Basic category and a combination of walk/jog in the Maintenance category. This is because weight-bearing activities are also associated with a higher incidence of injury. Therefore, those in the basic category, or those who are overweight or have arthritis, should begin with minimal weight-bearing activities.

Frequency

We use one week as a basis for determining the number of times you perform aerobic exercise. Adults need rest between workouts for the body to recover, and, if you're less fit, you need an even greater interval of time to recover. Therefore, I recommend those in the Basic category to start out two to three times a week. For those of you in the Maintenance category, three times a week. For the Experienced, start with three times a week and then slowly increase. A good idea is to alternate weight training with your aerobic activity to keep active and allow your body to recover by working out different muscle groups.

Intensity

Intensity is the component of your aerobics prescription that has the greatest potential for injury. For this reason, it is imperative that you continuously monitor your pulse and keep it near your training heart rate. Adjust the fitness factor as you calculate your proper THR. Those in the Basic category should begin with 50-70% of their max HR. Notice that you utilize the lowest factor, 50-60%, when doing aquatic or bicycle exercises. In these activities, you are not using as much muscle mass and/or are not carrying your total body weight. Consequently, there is not as much demand on your cardiovascular system. If you targeted a higher training heart rate you would actually be taxing your body more, or, in other words, be working out at a much higher intensity. Since intensity is associated with a higher risk, this would be a dangerous practice. As your aerobic fitness level improves, you can increase your intensity by multiplying by a larger fitness factor. For example, if you are in the Maintenance category, use a fitness factor of 70-80%, and in the Experienced category, a fitness factor of 80-85%.

NOTE:
Intensity is the component of your aerobics prescription that has the greatest potential for injury.

Time

The time, or duration, of your workout also varies with your aerobic fitness category. For those of you in the Basic category, your workout should be 15 to 20 minutes. If you are in the Maintenance category, you may increase that time to 30 minutes. If you're in the Experienced group, exercise for 30-60 minutes. If you want to achieve general all around aerobic conditioning, your goal should be an average of 30 minutes, three to four times a week. Remember, that you must exercise with 30 minutes of a sustained heart rate near your THR. For most people, this is enough time to get into true aerobic metabolism which means they are burning fat. Don't forget to add 20 to 40 minutes for the warm-up, cool-down, and the stretching phases, as discussed above. Thus, if your actual aerobics phase is 30 minutes your total session may exceed an hour.

Progression

Strictly speaking, I define progression as an increase in the <u>duration</u> of your aerobic phase of exercise. Keep in mind that slow, consistent progression prevents injury. If you are in the Basic category, increase your duration by 5% only after two weeks of stable exercise. If you are in the Maintenance category, you can increase by 5% after one week and 10% if in the Experienced category. You may be surprised to find that this is a small increase. For example, if your aerobic session is 30 minutes, a 5% increase adds only one and one half minutes to your workout. This may seem like a slow progression, but it's safe!

Making it Work for You

The beauty of this prescription system is that you can vary any one or more of these components and compensate by adjusting the remaining ones. For example, if you experience discomfort working in your selected training heart rate zone, you could <u>decrease</u> the intensity and <u>increase</u> the time. You would still achieve the same weekly benefit. Or, if there is a period when you cannot afford to devote so much time to your exercise routine, <u>decrease</u> the time and <u>increase</u> the frequency and/or intensity. By increasing some and decreasing other components of the prescription, the net result of your exercise will be the same.

Keep in mind, however, the most common cause of injury during exercise is high intensity, followed by frequency and then time. Time efficient routines revolving around periodic high intensity workouts of short duration lead to more injury, even though they may be convenient to the demands of your daily life. The safest routine builds around periodic, low intensity workouts of long duration, such as frequent long, slow walks. As you gain experience, you will be able to modify your own aerobic exercise prescription, adjusting your modality, frequency, intensity, time and progression.

NOTE:
The safest routine builds around periodic, low intensity workouts of long duration...

Table 2.12
GUIDELINES TO BEGIN AN AEROBIC ACTIVITY PROGRAM

	Basic	Maintenance	Experienced
Modality Type of Exercise	1. Aquatic Exercise 2. Swimming 3. Stationary Bicycle 4. Stationary Rowing 5. Trampoline 6. Dancing 7. Walking	1. Stair Stepper 2. Stair Climber 3. Stationary Skiing 4. Rowing 5. Hiking 6. Walk/Jog 7. Low Impact Aerobics	1. Skating 2. Roller Blading 3. Skipping Rope 4. Running 5. High Impact Aerobics
Frequency Days/Week	2-3	3	>3
Intensity % of Max HR	Aquatic/Bicycle 50-60% Others 60-70%	70-80%	80-85%
Time Minutes	15-20	30	>30
Progression % Increase in Time	5% every 2 weeks	5% per week	10% per week

Resources

As I mentioned previously, I believe the physical component, Body, is the most reasonable entry point into the model of total well being for the average American. Through physical activity you can learn how to find the movement into total well being . . . the movement that will help you integrate, then balance your Body, Mind and Spirit. That is why I'm writing **Total Well Being Through Physical Fitness**, the first in a series of companion manuals to this book (1). The manual will give you step by step instructions on how to assess your own fitness level, to exercise properly, and create your own personalized exercise prescription. You will do this using techniques that have been defined and tested by thousands of adults in medical environments where they have learned how to exercise properly and safely!

3 NUTRITION

Introduction

There have been thousands of books written on the subject of nutrition and diet . . . books that can provide you with invaluable information if you know how to use them. This chapter provides you with the knowledge you need in order to make informed choices about which of the resources on nutrition is best for you.

NOTE:
"Do not live to eat, but eat that you may live."

Dionysius of Halicarnassus, 8 B.C.

Diet and Nutrition

The terms diet and nutrition are frequently confused. For instance, we often hear the misleading statement that "diets don't work." Webster defines diet as "food and drink regularly provided or consumed." Since all of us eat and drink, we have diets that work, but in varying degrees from healthy to unhealthy.

Nutrition is defined as "the sum of the processes by which an animal takes in and utilizes food." In other words, nutrition is the process by which we use our diets to gain nourishment. Therefore, you can have good or bad nutrition based upon your good or bad diet, and the consequences are demonstrated by the health of your body.

The Nutrition Spectrum

When looking at nutrition, I refer to what I call the Nutrition Spectrum.

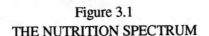

Figure 3.1
THE NUTRITION SPECTRUM

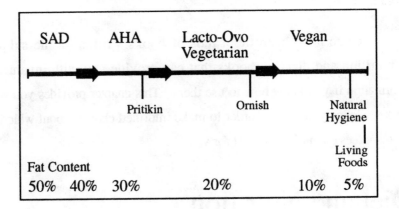

This spectrum starts on the left side with "SAD," which stands for the Standard American Diet and represents nutrition having the worst impact on our health. On the far right side, the spectrum ends with the "Vegan" diet, which is the ultimate in nutrition. In between are two other types of nutrition, including "AHA," the American Heart Association Diet, and the Lacto-Ovo-Vegetarian diet. Then, there are two subsets of vegan nutrition, Natural Hygiene and Living Foods.

Notice that the percentage of fat in our diets decreases as we move from the left (worst) to the right (best) across the nutrition spectrum. That, in and of itself, says a lot! Of all the nutrients we take in through our diets . . . carbohydrates, protein, fats, minerals, vitamins and water . . . fat has the most adverse effect on our health. The best way for us to understand why the diets at the right represent optimal nutrition is to look at each of the diets in the nutrition spectrum.

The Standard American Diet

The Standard American Diet, which most Americans eat, consists of highly refined, low fiber foods with an average of 40 to 50% fat! This explains why a recent, heavily publicized study describes fully one third of Americans as seriously overweight.[1] Over the years, a number of factors have converged to influence why we consider this unhealthy diet to be "normal." To a great extent, these factors stem from our affluence as a nation and our increasingly fast paced lives. Fat truly is the plague of opulence.

NOTE:
Fat is a poison!

Commercial food interests ply upon our lifestyles, selling us cost, convenience and taste with sophisticated marketing techniques to convince us to buy their products. The standards of the average American diet include fatty foods such as potato chips, french fries, ice cream, dairy products and hamburgers. Even "foreign foods" such as Tex Mex, Chinese and pizza are incredibly loaded with fat.

As a child, I remember that fat was a precious commodity. The most desired and expensive part of milk was the cream layered on top of the bottle. It was considered a special treat to have a bowl of cereal sprinkled with lots of sugar and filled to the brim with pure cream. Meat was also valued in terms of its fat content so that marbled steak was considered the best and, of course, the most expensive cut. Today, our nutritional values haven't changed as much as we might think.

Even with all the scientific research and publicity telling us how unhealthy a highly refined, high fat, low fiber diet is, we are still a nation that craves the Standard American Diet. Many of us simply ignore the facts, associating this diet with disease. In fact, most of us have no idea how much fat, sugar and salt we consume. We are oblivious to the paucity of fruits and vegetables we eat.

Yet, taken as a whole, the scientific literature shows that optimal health can be achieved from diets toward the right of the Nutrition Spectrum . . . an emphasis on a generous intake of fruits and vegetables.[2] Unquestionably, highly processed foods, high in animal fat, low in fiber and lacking vegetarian principles, are positively correlated with:

> **Heart Disease**[3]
> **High Blood Pressure**[4]
> **Cancer**[5]:
>> **Colon Cancer**[6,.7]
>> **Breast Cancer**[8]
>> **Prostate Cancer**[9]
>> **Oral Cavity, Larynx, Pancreas, Bladder and Cervical Cancer**[10, 11]
> **Arthritis**[12]
> **Cataracts**[13]

It is well known that **Obesity**, usually associated with dietary fat,[14,15] reduces life span. And, the greatest longevity is found in those whose weight is either below the average of the population under consideration,[16] or below relative weights by at least 10%[17] or 20%[18] of the US average. Finally, repeated studies show that **Adult Onset Diabetes** can be controlled with low fat diets.[19]

As you can clearly see, the Standard American Diet, with its high animal FAT and low vegetarian food content, is killing us. Fat is a poison! I urge you to find further information and references on the relationship between disease and diets high in fat. One such source is Marc Sorenson's book, **MegaHealth** (1).

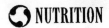

Animal Fat Versus Plant Oils

As one who is committed to exercise, the relationship of animal fat to inflammation is of special concern to me. Animal fats contain arachidonic acid, among other fatty acids. Arachidonic acid stimulates our cells to produce and release a chemical mediator called prostaglandin II. This sets in motion the inflammatory cascade that affects our joints, ligaments, tendons and muscles. Therefore, a diet high in animal fat is a hotbed for turning those minor strains and sprains into major aches and pains.

Interestingly enough, plant oils contain linolenic and linoleic fatty acids. These two fatty acids are what we call essential, since we can't make them ourselves. Furthermore, these fatty acids stimulate prostaglandin I, which <u>blocks</u> the inflammatory chain reaction. By avoiding animal fats and increasing your intake of plant oils by eating more vegetables, you will reduce those aggravating aches and pains associated with physical activity.

NOTE:
By avoiding animal fats . . . you will reduce those aggravating aches and pains associated with physical activity.

Sluggish Blood

Diets high in fat also cause our blood cells to clump together, which inhibits the flow of blood through your arteries. This compounds the problem of atherosclerosis, that I've already discussed, by further reducing the delivery of nutrients to our cells. A fatty diet delivers a double whammy to our circulatory systems. First, it contributes to plaque formation in our arteries and, then, creates sluggish blood flow as our blood cells clump together.

We Still Eat Fat

Despite all the information against fat, most Americans still eat many of their meals at fast food chains offering greasy hamburgers, french fries and deep fried chicken. A good example of our insistence on self-deception is the popularity of nuggets of chicken sold in fast food restaurants and supermarkets under the guise of a healthy chicken-based food choice. These morsels are composed of ground up chicken meat, often combined with fat scraped from the inside of the skin, then coated with crumbs, and deep fried in grease. So, what do we end up with? . . . Little fat balls!

When dipped in ketchup, which is composed of sugar, salt, vinegar and a little tomato paste, the devastating results are clear . . . sugar and fat - period! Once, when my children ate these chicken nuggets in our air conditioned kitchen, I noticed what was left on their plates when they were finished eating. The remaining little fat balls had all turned white; exactly like the congealed grease left over from frying bacon!

Dieting

NOTE:
Excess fat in our diet has contributed to an American epidemic of obesity . . .

Excess fat in the Standard American Diet has contributed to an American epidemic of obesity which, in turn, prompts millions of us to diet. Commonly, dieting is considered to be a plan where you restrict the calories you eat in order to lose weight. This is where we get the idea that "diets don't work," because, in the end, they don't.

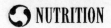

Diets Do Not Work Long-Term

Diets, especially the so called very low calorie diets of 800 Calories or less, do not work <u>long</u>-<u>term</u> for most people. Initially, there is a remarkable weight loss, decrease in blood cholesterol levels, reversal of diabetes and, often a feeling that borders on euphoria. In one of the best medically monitored programs, which also incorporates behavior modification and exercise, approximately 50% of the patients maintained their weight loss after two years.[20] However, studies from other programs show that five years after their initial weight loss, over 95% of dieters regain all their weight plus more.[21]

If you commit to a very low calorie diet to achieve a rapid weight loss, or for whatever reason, make sure it is monitored by a physician, incorporates a behavior modification and exercise component and provides for long term support. I've asked patients who have maintained their weight loss for up to two and three years what accounts for their success. Invariably, they respond with the same three answers; 1) regular exercise, 2) continual record keeping, or some other form of accountability and 3) attendance at maintenance or other support programs.

Why do most people have such a difficult time losing weight and keeping it off? Why is almost everyone you know on some kind of a "secret" diet, feeling guilty about what they eat and unhappy about how they look? In addition to the fact that most people diet for looks and not health, there are a variety of reasons diets don't work.

> **NOTE:**
> *. . . over 95%
> of dieters
> regain all
> their weight
> plus more.*

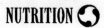

Why Don't Diets Work?

First, people generally eat in response to "stress." This type of "binge" eating cannot be eliminated by simply going on a diet. From my experiences as a physician dealing with weight loss programs, I conclude that the underlying psychological issues causing us to respond to stress by eating must be addressed along with any attempt to successfully lose and maintain weight loss. I'll discuss this further in Chapter 4, "Mental and Spiritual Fitness."

Secondly, the pressures of society <u>against</u> proper eating and nutrition must be dealt with by anyone desiring to lose weight and maintain his or her weight loss. To benefit from the opulence and freedoms of our society, we need to assume personal responsibility to eat a healthy diet. Successful "dieting" takes a commitment that most people can make if they are properly motivated. We <u>can</u> be successful in maintaining proper nutrition and, therefore, weight management by learning how to shop for food wisely . . . how to prepare healthy food . . . and how to make healthy food choices when we eat out. Then, we need to incorporate healthy attitudes and exercise to round out our lifestyle changes. Successful weight management is not changing our <u>diets</u>, it's changing our <u>lifestyles</u>!

A third reason dieters aren't successful has to do with our bodies' adjustment to low calorie diets or, in physiological terms, starvation. For years, I have managed patients who successfully lost weight on very low calorie diets. Unfortunately, for any or all of the reasons mentioned here, many of them put their weight back on.

For example, many of my patients lost weight prior to the fall of 1992. Then, Hurricane Andrew hit. This disaster, along with its incredible

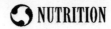

acute trauma and long term stresses, was as close to a legitimate excuse as one could find for improper eating and weight gain. When these once successful dieters re-entered the program, even after three years, their weight would not come off as it had originally, despite the fact that they adhered to the same caloric restricted diet. Clearly, our metabolic rates decrease with weight loss, although the rate is not abnormally below that expected from our concomitant loss of body tissue.[22] Based upon experiences like those above, however, I suspect that repeated bouts of weight loss lower our metabolic rates lower and for longer periods of time with each weight loss cycle. Moreover, I believe this "starvation mode" is imprinted in our bodies, making it more difficult to lose weight each time we cycle through a caloric restricted diet.

Lastly, emphasis on the number of calories in foods and calorie counting is, at best, inaccurate and unreliable. Simply calculating the <u>percent</u> of <u>fat</u> in our food is an easier and more pragmatic approach to determining what food we should eat. This method addresses the issues of the harmful effects of fat, as well as it's higher caloric content. Let's see why calorie counting doesn't work and counting percent fat does.

NOTE:
Simply calculating the <u>percent</u> <u>of fat</u> in our food is an easier and more pragmatic approach to determining what food we should eat.

Caloric Expenditure

Most of us count calories and exercise to help control our weight. Calories are simply a measurement of how much energy we get from our food. For example, the following represents the number of calories in each of the three food categories:

Carbohydrates	4 calories per gram
Proteins	4 calories per gram
Fats	9 calories per gram

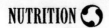

This simple comparison tells us something right off the bat. Fat has twice as many calories as sugar (carbohydrates) or protein. In fact, you could totally replace all the "diet" books on the shelves of every book store with one sign, ⊘FAT . That's being a bit facetious because we must take in essential fatty acids, but we will get all we need with proper nutrition!

Have you ever noticed that sometimes "calorie" is written or abbreviated with a capital "C" even in the middle of a sentence? The reason for this is that calories are derived from grams of food. One gram is a tiny amount . . . much less than a thimbleful. Because it's so small, scientists simply multiply everything by 1,000 which equals a *kilo*. That turns these units into *kilo*grams and *kilo*calories, the later of which is typically abbreviated with a capital "C". Thus, a calorie equals one calorie while a Calorie (Cal) equals 1,000 calories.

How Many Calories Do You Burn in a Day?

NOTE:

To determine your resting metabolic rate, multiply your weight by 11.

You can easily estimate your daily caloric expenditure by utilizing simple formulas. First, determine your resting metabolic rate or the number of Calories you would burn if you just sat in a chair all day. To do this, multiply your weight in pounds by 11.

Weight ▨▨▨ (pounds) x 11 = ▨▨▨ Cal

Since you do more than sit all day, you need to add a certain number of Calories to account for your daily level of activity. So, add 400 if your life is basically sedentary, 600 if you lead a moderately active life, and 800 if you are very active; for example, if you perform heavy labor, walk a lot, or climb with heavy loads. This gives you your daily metabolic rate. Later, there will be a place for you to add Calories from planned exercise.

Fill in the following formulas to estimate your Daily Metabolic Rate.

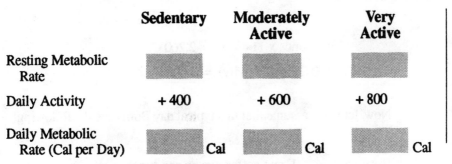

	Sedentary	Moderately Active	Very Active
Resting Metabolic Rate			
Daily Activity	+ 400	+ 600	+ 800
Daily Metabolic Rate (Cal per Day)	Cal	Cal	Cal

NOTE:
To determine your daily metabolic rate, add 400, 600 or 800 Calories depending on your activity level.

Your estimated Daily Metabolic Rate simply means that if you eat food equal to the number of Calories you expend each day, you will stay at your same weight. If you eat fewer Calories, you will lose weight, and if you eat more, you will gain weight. Where does the weight go? You guessed it. For men it's around their middle, and for women it's in their buttocks and thighs.

How Many Calories Do You Take in a Day?

Now that you know how many Calories you <u>expend</u> in an average day, how do you suppose you fare in balancing those against the number of Calories you <u>take in</u> each day? In other words, how's your weight?

For example, let's take someone who is sedentary and weighs 200 pounds. I'll use these same numbers throughout the chapter for other sample calculations, so let's give this phantom person a name . . . like Boris. Remember now, Boris is a sedentary person who weighs 200 pounds.

According to our formulas above, Boris has a Daily Metabolic Rate of 2,600 Cal.

$$200 \text{ pounds} \times 11 = 2,200 \text{ Calories}$$
$$+ 400 \text{ (Daily Activity)} = 2,600 \text{ Calories}$$

Now, let's just assume that in a typical day Boris eats the following:

Breakfast:

1	cup coffee, cream and sugar	40
1	cup OJ	80
2	scrambled eggs	190
2	sausage links	200
2	slices wheat toast	140
2	tablespoons margarine	90
2	teaspoons jelly	40
	Total	780

That may be a big breakfast for some, so I'll skip the "coffee" break and move right on to lunch.

Lunch:

1	cup mushroom soup	200
12	goldfish crackers	30
1	BLT sandwich	455
1	piece banana cream pie	300
	Total	985

Mind you, that's a small piece of banana cream pie. Next, let's assume Boris had a terrible day at work and, upon arriving home, the kids insist on going out to their favorite fast food restaurant. First, this requires a few moments of relaxation with a "drink". . . notice, it's with "diet" soda.

Dinner:	2 rum & diet sodas	240
	1 triple burger	850
	1 large fries	330
	1 medium chocolate shake	390
	Total	1,810

TOTAL CALORIES   3,575!

When I go through this scenario, some people resist, claiming that they would never eat so much, especially for breakfast and lunch. But, what about those "coffee" breaks or late night snacks of potato chips, pretzels or that hot fudge sundae? They would easily go for another 1,000 Calories.

So, let's see how Boris fares in the weight department:

Total Calories In	3,750
Total Calories Out	2,600
Total Calories to Fat	1,150

Despite the enormous number of calories in-versus-the calories out, some of my patients simply refuse to give up their favorite foods, especially those late night snacks. They say, "Well, I'll just start exercising and burn off those extra calories that I ate." Let's see how that works.

NOTE:
"Well, I'll just start exercising and burn off those extra calories that I ate."

How Many Calories Do You Burn with Exercise?

Take a look at the activities listed in Table 3.1. Choose the activities that might interest you and determine the number of Calories you would burn from that activity. The middle column displays the number of Calories burned in <u>one solid hour</u> of activity, expressed as Cal/hr. Keep in mind that these are only rough estimates. There are a lot of variables that could interfere with trying to pre-determine the way you would do the same activity. Such variables might include the intensity of the workout, the type of equipment used, the location of your exercise, weather conditions, etc.

In addition, notice that each value is based upon the amount of energy required for a 170 pound person. If you weigh less, it wouldn't take as much energy to perform that activity, since you wouldn't be pushing and pulling as many pounds. If you weigh more, you would burn more Calories. Therefore, as directed in the right-hand column, divide 170 into your weight and multiply that whole number or fraction by the Cal/hr for that activity. This will give you the number of Calories you would burn based upon your body weight.

One more thing to remember, however, is that these values are for one solid, consistent hour of activity. You may need to make an adjustment, depending upon how long you exercise. For example, you would halve the number of Calories for a 30 minute exercise session.

Let's assume that Boris has decided to exercise and chooses walking for 30 minutes. His calculations would go like this:

Walking (from Table 3.1)	= 222 Cal/hr
200 pounds ÷ 170	= 1.2 (weight adjustment factor)
1.2 x 222 Cal/hr	= 266 Cal/hr
266 Cal/hr ÷ 0.5 hr	= 133 Calories per walking 30 min

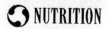

Table 3.1
CALORIC EXPENDITURE FOR A VARIETY OF ACTIVITIES*

Activity	Cal/hr (For a 170 lb person)	Your Cal/hr (Your Wt ÷ 170x middle column)
Canoeing, leisure (2.5 mph)	204	
Walking, 2 mph	222	
Golf, walking (4-some)	276	
Dancing, modern (moderate)	282	
Baseball	300	
Bicycling, 5.5 mph (11 min/mile)	306	
Boxing, sparring	336	
Dancing, modern (vigorous)	384	
Swimming, pleasure (25 yds/min)	408	
Walking, 4.5 mph (13 min/mile)	450	
Tennis, recreational	468	
Baketball, moderate	474	
Weight Training	534	
Skiing, downhill	654	
Rope Skipping, 809/min	672	
Racquetball	678	
Swimming, crawl (50 yds/min)	720	
Running, 5.5 mph (11 min/mile)	726	
Skiing, cross country (5 mph)	792	
Running 7 mph (8.5 min/mile)	942	

*Taken from: Stokes, R., et al. **Fitness, the New Wave**. Hunter Textbooks, Inc., Winston-Salem, NC. 1988; 230-232.

Marathon Runners - How Do They Do It?

This brings me to an intriguing question that I asked myself early on in my sports medicine practice. Again and again, I would witness skinny young men and women run a 26.2 mile marathon. I knew that endurance running required the burning of fat, but I couldn't figure out where they hid all that fat to get enough energy to keep going. You can learn a lot from this, so, I'd like you to guess at the following questions:

1. How many calories does it take to run one mile Cal

2. How many calories are there in one pound of fat? ▢ Cal

Now, I've spent a lot of time rearranging this text so that the answers appear on the next page. Don't cheat by looking across the page for the solution! Just make a guess. There's a valuable lesson to be learned here. OK, did you guess? . . . If not try again.

1. How many calories does it take to run one mile? ▢ Cal

2. How many calories are there in one pound of fat? ▢ Cal

Now, you may go to the next page.

1 mile	=	100 Cal
1 pound of fat	=	3,500 Cal
1 marathon	=	2,600 Cal

It takes less than one pound of fat to run a marathon! Amazing, isn't it?

Calories In, Calories Out - or "Easy Come, Hard to Go"

Based upon the information and the mental exercises above, most people accept that we consume calories far in excess to those which we expend in a typical day. However, most people are surprised at how few calories we burn with exercise.

Actually, exercise helps us maintain a proper body composition in another way. As I discussed in Chapter 2, with exercise we gain muscle mass, which is much more metabolically active than fat. This increases the metabolic rate so our bodies burn more calories at rest. However, muscle weighs about twice as much as fat so the total body weight may not reflect the improved body composition. This is one of the reasons that your % body fat is a much better indicator of your body composition than total body weight.

The above information, especially Table 3.1, also points out that you gain the maximum benefit from aerobic activity with sustained exercise. This burns fat, which in and of itself is a miracle substance.

NOTE:
. . . we consume calories far in excess to those which we expend in a typical day.

Fat: Easy Come/Easy Go

Despite the 1990's war on fat, it is one of the many miracles of our bodies. Unused fragments of carbohydrates, proteins and fats that we take in automatically and easily flow thorough metabolic pathways into fat storage. When the need arises, fat is just as easily broken down at little energy cost to the body. Moreover, the breakdown products of fat lead directly into a metabolic pathway where, in the presence of oxygen, enormous amounts of energy are produced. This means that fat is a readily accessible and an incredibly concentrated storage form of calories.

However, there is a common sense argument that makes fat an even more astonishing creation. Fat is an oil, meaning that it doesn't mix with water. Think about it. If we stored the same amount of concentrated energy that we find in fat in a water soluble substance, our bodies would be so overloaded with water . . . so heavy . . . that we would not be able to walk on land! Primitive man surely benefited from this miracle substance by using periods of feast to store up energy for periods of famine. In our affluent society, however, it's up to us to be wise and not pay the consequences of over indulgent eating habits. We can count calories . . . or perhaps there is a better way.

Percent of Fat Content in Food

Counting Calories is plagued with pitfalls. I've already mentioned how we underestimate the volume of food we eat and, therefore, the number of Calories we consume based on tables that express Caloric food values in ounces. It's even more complex because oils utilized in food preparation can throw off caloric intake by ten-fold!

Furthermore, estimating caloric expenditure is fraught with inaccuracies. I'll bet that you questioned some of the Caloric expenditure values in Table 3.1 above. Just think of all the variables that affect such estimates associated with exercise, such as your metabolism, body composition (not just total body weight) and all of the environmental conditions which I mentioned earlier.

However, since fat accounts for twice the calories of other foods and is associated with numerous diseases, let's just focus on the amount of fat we take in. In fact, determining the fat content of food is the newest and easiest approach to counting "Calories." If we eat foods that have a fat content of 10% to 20% or less, we couldn't possibly eat enough bulk to yield the extra Calories to gain weight! The FDA is now making it easy to determine % fat in food by mandating uniform labeling for all packaged food. Simply look at the Nutrition Facts panel on the package of any food you have in your house to see what I mean.

Let's take a look at the label on a medium size bag of "New and Improved," 40% Less Fat Potato Chips. I've omitted the labeled Calories from Fat until you do the calculation.

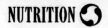

Nutrition Facts

Serving Size 1 oz. (28g/about 20 chips)
Servings Per Container about 5

Amount Per Serving

Calories 130	Calories from Fat

	% Daily Value
Total Fat 6g	9%
Saturated Fat 1g	5%
Cholesterol 0mg	0%
Sodium 5mg	0%
Total Carbohydrate 17g	3%
Dietary Fiber 1g	4%
Sugars 0g	
Protein 2g	

Now, using this label, here are the steps to determine Calories from fat:

1. Identify how many grams of fat there are per serving.
2. Multiply this number by 9 to get the number of fat Calories per serving.
3. Then, divide by the total number of Calories per serving.
4. Lastly, multiply by 100 to get the %.

Here's how to do the simple arithmetic:

1. Grams of Fat per Serving   =   6
2. Multiply by 9 (Calories per 1 gram Fat) =   54
3. Divide by Calories per Serving (130)   =   .42
4. Multiply by 100   =   42% Cal from Fat!

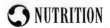

A healthy diet has less than 20% fat or, even better, less than 10% fat. An excellent way to practice optimal nutrition is to avoid eating foods that have more than 10% fat calories. This would certainly preclude these "40% less fat" chips. By the way, if you can't eat just one potato chip, and might just eat the whole bag, that's 650 Calories and 30 grams of fat!

Number of Grams of Fat Per Day

Another way to address the amount of fat in our diets by using the Nutrition Facts panel, is to determine the number of grams of fat we should consume each day. Simply calculate your Daily Calories (page 125) and then multiply by whatever you want your % fat intake to be, for example 15%. This gives you the number of daily fat calories you're allowed. Then divide by 9 to get the number of grams of fat.

Let us use Boris as an example. But first, congratulations are in order! Boris has taken up walking, so his Daily Metabolic Rate is now 2,800 Calories. Furthermore, since he's feeling so much better he made the commitment to healthy nutrition by eating a 15% fat diet. His calculations would go like this:

2,800 Daily Calories x 15%   = 420 Fat Calories

420 Fat Calories ÷ 9 grams/Cal   = 47 grams of Fat

Seem impossible? Lots of people have come alive with good nutrition. Read on and you'll see that you can do it too!

The American Heart Association Diet

Over the past ten years our awareness of good-versus-bad nutrition has improved. Our medical societies have become more concerned and have made recommendations to decrease the amount of fat in our diets. As we continue along the nutrition spectrum, we come to the American Heart Association's recommendations that a "good" diet should decrease the amount of fat to 30%. In essence, this diet allows meats, fish, fowl and dairy products, along with the standard fare, but with slightly reduced fat content. This is a move in the right direction, but falls far short of optimal nutrition.

For example, population studies have shown a <u>reduced</u> incidence of breast cancer in women who eat a vegetarian diet.[23] Yet, a recent study claimed that a low fat diet did not lower the rate of breast cancer in women followed over three years.[24] What was their low fat diet? The recommended AHA 30% fat diet!

Characteristically, the medical establishment is conservative and slow to respond to change. We need a "watch dog" organization to shield us against charlatans in the critically important arena dealing with our health and welfare. However, there is enough credible scientific and basic biological information for us to take action in moving to the right of the spectrum . . . away from the American Heart Association diet toward even more optimal nutrition. Another way to justify this approach is from the perspective of basic human anatomy, physiology and biochemistry.

Humans Are Herbivores

By nature, human beings are herbivores. Let's start out at the beginning of the digestive tract and see how our anatomy and physiology support this concept, Table 3.2.

Our Teeth

For example, our teeth, particularly our canines, are not at all like the longer pointed teeth of carnivores such as tigers or wolves. These animals must tear through the thick hides of animals to feed. Moreover, unlike the jaws of carnivores which lock in place and can move only up and down, we can move our jaws from side to side similar to plant chewing animals. In fact, we are much closer in chewing motions to the cud chewing ruminants . . . herbivores like cows, goats or deer.

Our Salivary Juices

We secrete two digestive enzymes in our mouths called amylase and lipase. Amylase digests starch, and if we chewed slowly and kept the food in our mouths for a long enough period of time, the amylase would digest 75% of all of the starch we consume. Lipase is an enzyme that begins the breakdown of fats. It is noteworthy that both of these enzymes break down food components which we, as animals, store as energy for later use. There are no enzymes in our mouths, however, that breaks down protein, the main component of meat.

Our Stomachs

Continuing down the digestive tract to our stomachs, we see that it is designed to digest only protein. As protein enters our stomachs it stimulates the release of concentrated hydrochloric acid from the stomach wall. The acid, in turn, stimulates the production of an enzyme that breaks down the protein into simpler more easily absorbed molecules.

When we eat dense protein foods, such as meat and dairy products, excessive amounts of acid are secreted. These stomach juices are so caustic that if you were to put your finger in them you would come up with nothing but a stub! Indigestion, heartburn and ulcers, the most common intestinal disorders in our society today, result from consuming too much protein and excessive acid formation. Indeed, the number one selling prescription drug in America is a medication that temporarily blocks the synthesis of stomach acid.

Our Intestines

Our intestines are what I call the "outside inside us." That is, the lumen of our guts contains the world that we swallow, including any disease producing organisms, allergens and poisons, plus an intricately balanced population of over 400 species of bacteria. This amazing organ, then, must play a dual role of keeping out the undesirable organisms and poisons, fending off the allergens, while, simultaneously, selectively allowing the essential nutrients in.

Our intestines are approximately seven times our body length in comparison to a carnivore's, which is approximately three times its body length. Meat eaters have shorter intestines so they can more rapidly evacuate the decaying breakdown products of the flesh they eat. We pay a price by eating meat, because it decays or putrefies as it lumbers through our much longer intestines.

Putrefaction

When we eat meat, we usually eat too much at one time <u>and</u> do not chew it thoroughly. Consequently, our intestinal juices can't completely digest it, and partially digested pieces of meat pass into the large intestine, called the colon. This upsets the delicate balance of bacteria in our colons which leads to decay or putrefaction, see Figure 3.2.

Putrefaction of protein and fat produces biological chemicals that are toxic to our bodies. Some of these toxins are carcinogenic, meaning that they may produce cancer, which could explain the link between meat eaters and their higher incidence of colon cancer.[25] Most of the toxins are eliminated with our stool, but, when in excess, they may be reabsorbed back into our blood streams. They circulate to our livers where they are detoxified and excreted through our kidneys. However, a flood of toxins can overload the liver and pass right on through to the rest of our bodies. These toxins can then produce a plethora of symptoms such as headaches, muscle aches and pains, fatigue, bad breath, allergies and just plain not feeling well.

This describes the "unwell" population on the Health Continuum. Note, that by changing lifestyle . . . practicing true preventive medicine by modifying their nutrition . . . these people could move toward total well being.

Fiber Not Meat

One way to avoid the production of these toxins is to avoid eating meat and to eat lots of fiber. Fiber acts as a barrier against the absorption of toxins and speeds up the movement of these products through the colon. Meat-eating carnivores don't experience these problems because the meat products they eat are excreted quicker from their shorter intestines before toxic build-up occurs. Once again, we see how our anatomy is designed for vegetarian foods, rather than meats.

Table 3.2
HUMANS ARE HERBIVORES
Based Upon Our Anatomy and Physiology

Principle	Carnivores	Humans
Teeth	Tearing Canines	Chewing Molars
Jaws	Locked, Up and Down	Side to Side
Salivary Enzymes		Carbohydrate and Fat Digesting
Protein Digestion	Adapted	Excess Acid Produces Ulcers
Intestine	3 x Body Length	7 x Body Length
Putrification	Minimal	Excessive Unless Vegetarian

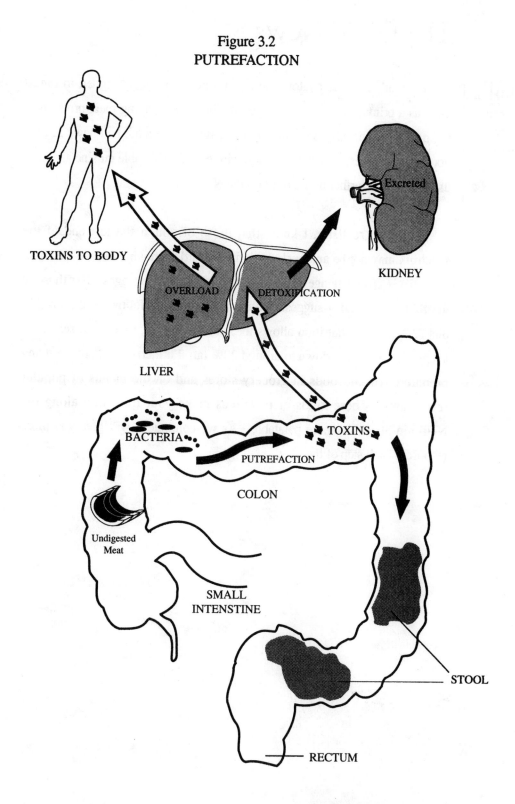

Figure 3.2
PUTREFACTION

The Good News

NOTE:

"The absurd man is he who never changes."

Auguste Barthélémy, 1830

Our intestinal anatomy and physiology are <u>not</u> designed to digest meat as a primary food. In addition, the fat accompanying meat products is harmful to our health, as previously discussed. That's the bad news . . . the good news is, there is better nutrition with equally palatable cuisine ahead of us as we move further to the right on the Nutrition Spectrum.

To be realistic, I know that those of you at the left end of the spectrum may not be anxiously looking forward to moving toward the right. And, that's OK. Change is a process which occurs in stages. For those at the SAD/AHA end, I suggest making a first step by following the Pritikin diet (2,3,4). This nutrition allows the same foods but, by careful selection, keeps the fat content down to around 20% fat. Furthermore, there are many prepared Pritikin foods in grocery stores and on the menus of popular restaurants. These kinds of resources make your transition along the Nutrition Spectrum more palatable. As we continue, I will give you more resources each step of the way.

The Lacto-Ovo-Vegetarian Diet

The lacto-ovo-vegetarian, or lacto-vegetarian diet for short, excludes meat, fish and poultry, but does include eggs and dairy products, such as milk, cheese, butter and yogurt. This diet, when carefully monitored, can be kept to 20% fat. Many lacto-vegetarian dishes can be prepared similar to the SAD/AHA diet providing tasty, yet healthier, cuisine. With a little education, you can select foods consistent with this nutrition when dining out. You can even move further into the lacto-vegetarian spectrum to keep your fat content to within 10%. Therefore, the lacto-vegetarian diet serves as an excellent <u>transition</u> as you move across the nutrition spectrum.

However the lacto-vegetarian diet is still lacking, since it does not avoid the conditions associated with animal fats, and because it still includes milk-based dairy products. There is growing evidence that animal proteins, such as those contained in milk, are unhealthy to humans.

NOTE:
The lacto-vegetarian diet serves as an excellent <u>transition</u> to optimal nutrition.

Why Not Milk?

Even before my research into the field of nutrition, I was curious about why humans drink milk when no other adult animal consumes milk. Not only that, but we consume milk from an entirely different species of animal. Throughout my years of study in biology and medicine, I have learned to appreciate the miracle of life. I have gained a spiritual reverence for nature that goes well beyond any other knowledge I've developed. It makes simple common sense to me that if other animals stop drinking their mother's milk upon maturation, we human animals should avoid it also.

In addition to this common sense argument, there is a basic biological concept that supports the fact that excessive protein, whether in meat or dairy products, is harmful to our health. Our entire metabolic machinery, including the metabolism of food and the production of energy, relies upon an interrelated series of chain reactions controlled by enzymes, plus a host of other support players called coenzymes, vitamins and minerals, Figure 3.3.

Figure 3.3
THE ROLE OF ENZYMES IN OUR METABOLIC MACHINERY

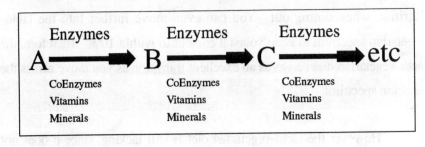

NOTE:

... enzymes are extremely sensitive to the proper acid/base balance in our bodies. Without proper balance our bodies' metabolism ʰᵘᵗ ᵈᵒʷⁿ

Enzymes are often described as the distinguishing feature between living and non-living forms because they drive the millions of chain ...tions in our bodies, which are basic to life. However, enzymes are :emely sensitive to the proper acid/base balance in our bodies. ...racteristically, we produce far more acids than bases. Stop a moment ...see if you can think of some acids in our bodies that harm us when we ...duce too much.

Did you consider lactic acid, a waste product built up in our muscles after prolonged exercise? How about uric acid, a by-product of rich foods that can lead to gout? What about excessive stomach acid producing indigestion and ulcers?

Protein, an Acid Producer

The largest source of acid production in our bodies is from protein. First, the sulfur and phosphorous in protein are converted into highly caustic sulfuric and phosphoric acids. However, the main source of protein-generated acids comes from the amino group which is a unique component of the amino acids that make up protein. Collectively, these acid loads can interfere with the entire functioning of our physiology by creating a hostile environment in which enzymes must function. It stands to reason that we should minimize our intake of protein . . . the biggest potential acid producer of anything we eat.

> **NOTE:**
>
> *Acids from protiein can interfere with our entire physiological function.*

Milk Protein and Allergies

Milk contains concentrated protein which is where we get the phrase "liquid meat." This used to be an argument for the value of milk. However, as you will see, we get an <u>excess</u> of protein in our diets which <u>decreases</u> the value of milk as a nutrient. When we ingest these foreign proteins, they often produce an allergic reaction. Our gastrointestinal tracts react to this allergy by leaking more of these ingested proteins into our systems which leads to allergies in other parts of our bodies.

For example, we may develop allergic reactions in our respiratory systems. When this occurs, the delicate linings in our sinuses, ears, and lungs become irritated. We get more viral and bacterial infections. Our bodies wall off these invaders with mucous in order for us to more easily get rid of them. Since our children eat and drink excessive amounts of dairy products, this helps to explain the ever increasing incidence of upper respiratory and ear problems they endure.

These allergic reactions can also cause asthma, seen predominately in children and adolescents. In adults, the allergic reactions may show up in joints, causing arthritic pain.

Milk Associated With Other Problems

NOTE:

With all of the problems associated with milk, it makes little sense to consume milk products derived from other animals.

The high fat, low fiber content of milk is also detrimental to our health. This is animal fat, just like meat, which is associated with atherosclerosis. Even milk labeled as "low fat" is misleading since its fat content is based upon the liquid volume of the milk, which is predominately water. When calculated according to its dry weight, low fat milk has 24-33% fat as calories.

Other concerns associated with milk consumption include its possible relationship to childhood diabetes mellitus[26], lymphatic organ cancers[27] and other cancers.[28] Moreover, many decry the potential metabolic effects of bovine growth hormone (BGH) which has recently been introduced in our milk supply.[29]

Another problem with dairy products has to do with milk sugar, lactose. Up to 40% of Caucasians and 90% of Blacks have a deficiency in the enzyme lactase that digests milk sugar. Undigested lactose causes abdominal discomfort, gas, bloating and diarrhea.

Therefore, from the biological, physiological, nutritional and medical standpoint, it makes little sense to consume milk from other animals. Moreover, there are healthy, delicious alternatives such as rice, soy and nut milks. These milks are far less allergenic, more easily digested, and contain far less saturated fat. I'll describe these alternatives further in the practical applications section of this chapter.

Intestinal Gas

The food we eat and the manner in which we eat it may produce intestinal gas. Gas is caused by three events: 1) air swallowing, 2) intestinal production from bacteria and 3) diffusion from blood. Air swallowing accounts for most of the gas in our stomachs and is mostly relieved by burping. Bacterial production of gas in our colons account for most of the gas which is passed per rectum. Absorption of gas from our blood plays a small role in producing intestinal gas, except in abnormal metabolic states.

Interestingly, bloating and abdominal distention are not caused by excessive gas, but rather from decreased intestinal motility. This suggests that those foods you think may be producing gas are, in reality, toxins that block the ability of muscles along your intestinal tract to move bowel components through your intestine.

Air Swallowing

You can minimize the amount of air you swallow by chewing your food slowly and completely. This decreases air swallowed with chunks of food, and it grinds the existing air out of the food you eat. You can also minimize air swallowing by not gulping liquids with or without meals and by cutting down on chewing gum.

Colon Gas

Under normal physiological conditions, we secrete enzymes into our small intestines that digest food particles into smaller and smaller molecules that are then absorbed into our blood streams. Only the cell wall of plants (cellulose) and other undigested fibers reach the colon, which, along with bacteria, form the bulk of our stool.

However, when undigested food reaches the colon, it is broken down by bacteria that results in gas production. Carbohydrates undergo the process of fermentation, while proteins and fats undergo putrefaction as discussed above.

NOTE:
Gas in the colon is produced when undigested food reaches the colon because we eat too much food at one sitting without chewing it completely.

One of the main reasons undigested food reaches the colon is because we eat too much food at one sitting without chewing it completely. In this case, chunks of food can't be thoroughly digested by the enzymes in the small intestine before they reach the colon. In other cases, people simply don't have the intestinal enzymes to digest certain foods, so they end up in the colon.

Milk Intolerance

As I mentioned previously, over half of our population is deficient in the intestinal enzyme lactase, which is needed to digest the sugar in milk (lactose). When these individuals eat dairy products, the milk sugar is fermented by intestinal and colon bacteria and produces varying degrees of gas, diarrhea and abdominal pain. "Lactaid" is an enzyme preparation that can be swallowed to help in the digestion of lactose which minimizes these symptoms. A better approach, for reasons I discussed earlier regarding milk, is simply to avoid dairy products altogether.

Beans

Some legumes, like beans, contain sugar in their cell wall which humans cannot digest by their intestinal enzymes. When this sugar reaches

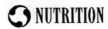

the colon, it is fermented by bacteria, producing the gas frequently associated with baked beans. This problem can be minimized by soaking beans for 12 hours and then letting them sprout to predigest the carbohydrate coat. You can also use a product called "Beano," which is an enzyme that digests the bean sugar before it reaches the colon.

Food Combining

Gas is also produced when certain food groups are introduced into our intestines together. One combination you could avoid is sugar, as in fruits, combined with protein, as in beans, or tofu. In the presence of intestinal bacteria, this combination sets up a fermentation mix analogous to the fermentation process used in making wine or beer. It is different, however, in that gas and vinegar are produced, rather than alcohol. You can learn more about food combining by reading the literature from the American Natural Hygiene Society (see Resources 12, 13).

Fiber

The colon contains millions of bacteria from hundreds of different species which normally live in a harmonious community. If this population becomes overgrown with certain species due to the presence of excessive undigested foods, these bacteria can produce excess gas of the odiferous type. Many of the toxins produced by putrefaction (refer back to Figure 3.2) are responsible for these gases. You can minimize this problem by avoiding the passage of undigested food particles into the colon as discussed above. In addition, a proper balance of bacteria can be maintained by moving the bowel contents along on a timely basis.

Generally speaking, this means having a soft formed bowel movement once a day. The most natural way to accomplish this is with a diet high in fiber. The SAD Fare, a diet high in protein and low in fiber, provides the colon with the very foods that encourage overgrowth of the bacteria that cause putrefaction and gas. Moreover, there is little fiber in this diet, which creates stagnation, further leading to gas production. You can correct this by turning toward a vegetarian diet, eating plenty of fiber or taking fiber supplements to keep the bowel contents moving regularly.

Many people who become gaseous at the outset of a vegetarian diet falsely blame the diet. In fact, once their colon bacteria adapt, they will have much less gas due to more fiber clearing the colon and revitalizing friendly bacteria.

In summary, Table 3.3 shows you ways to minimize intestinal gas.

Table 3.3
WAYS TO MINIMIZE EXCESS INTESTINAL GAS

1. Eat slowly and thoroughly chew your food.
2. Avoid gulping liquids and chewing gum.
3. Soak and sprout beans and/or use Beano with meals.
4. Minimize milk and dairy products and/or use lactaid.
5. Eat plenty of fiber or take fiber supplements.
6. Combine foods properly.

Making The Transition

I am now going to move along the nutrition spectrum into an area that may seem radical to some of you. Indeed, a few years ago, I thought vegetarianism was far out . . . that vegetarian diets went along with only hippies and flower children. Fortunately, "the times they are a changin'." Do you remember the disbelief when Nathan Pritikin proposed diets to prevent heart disease over ten years ago? Now, Pritikin foods are on the shelves of supermarkets and the menus of restaurants across the country. Based upon my own personal experience and what I see in the rapidly expanding field of nutritional science, I believe vegan and living food nutrition will be commonplace in the years to come.

Our country has been conducting an uncontrolled nutritional experiment on us by providing high fat, low fiber, highly refined, toxic-laden foods for our consumption. Look around you . . . we are the losers! Let's remember, however, that the food industry is consumer driven. It will apply its incredible talents and resources to give us what we demand. Take the "fortified foods" response decades ago, or the current "low fat" trend. The commercial foods industry is just that . . . commercial . . . it's up to us.

I know that making change is not easy. Some of you will take it in leaps and bounds, others in small increments. The point is, change! Wherever you are on the Nutrition Spectrum, take a step to the right. I've found that little steps make it easier and easier for me to take bigger steps. I occasionally back-slide, and then discover that the old food doesn't taste as good as I had thought, and I don't like feeling ill the next few days. It becomes easier and easier to stay on track.

NOTE:
"A journey of a thousand miles must begin with a single step."
Chinese Proverb

Little steps include moving from the SAD fare to the American Heart Association diet by reducing portion sizes of meat. A dear friend and colleague of mine, an endocrinologist, recently began to change his nutrition and now recommends the same for his patients. He advises people to use small amounts of meat as a "flavoring" in their main course, rather than large cuts occupying the center of their dish. Gradually move into Pritikin nutrition by replacing red meat with fish and fowl. Then, for those of you who have adopted lacto-vegetarian nutrition, move to a transition point between that and the vegan diet with Dean Ornish's program (5,6). Dr. Ornish has designed a cuisine equally as tasty as lacto-vegetarian foods, but he recommends only egg whites, skim milk and low fat yogurt. Otherwise, his dietary recommendations are strictly vegetarian. From there you can gradually move toward the ultimate in nutrition . . . the vegan concept.

The Vegan Diet

This diet includes fruits, vegetables, seeds, nuts and grains, either cooked or raw. The issue of cooked-versus-raw distinguishes whether it is Vegan or the sub set of diets, Natural Hygiene and Living Foods. We can maintain optimal nutrition and excellent cuisine by staying with a Vegan diet, especially if we maintain an 80% fresh and 20% cooked combination of vegetarian foods. The best way to come to grips with understanding the language of a vegan diet is to refer to a new classification of food groups proposed by Dr. Bernard (7,8).

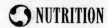

The Four Food Groups

This is a new classification which emphasizes the optimal vegan nutrition and includes fruits, vegetables, legumes and grains. These four food groups can be more fully understood by referring to Figure 3.4.

Figure 3.4
THE FOUR FOOD GROUPS OF A VEGAN DIET

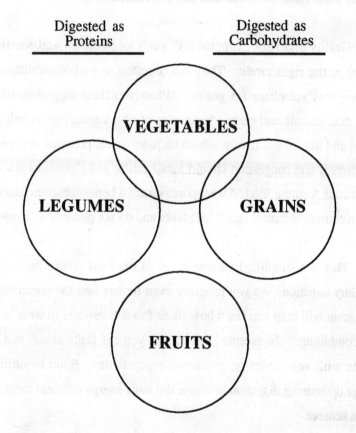

Digested as
Proteins

Digested as
Carbohydrates

Vegetables should form the staple of our nutrition since they provide all of the essential nutrients we need. In addition, they add fiber to our diets which creates buffers against toxic build-up in our colons, as discussed earlier, Figure 3.2.

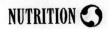

Fruits stand alone at the bottom of the diagram. Fruits provide valuable and unique contributions to our nutrition, but they contain sugar. Although not refined, fruit sugar (fructose) is metabolized the same way and, therefore, may cause the same problems as plain sugar. Remember, also, that tomatoes are frequently mistaken as a vegetable, but are really a fruit.

Legumes, such as beans, peas, seeds and nuts are included in the left circle. These foods are digested in the body as proteins, and so we may substitute these foods for meats and dairy products.

Grains and root "vegetables" such as potatoes and squash are included in the right circle. They are digested as carbohydrates, a term which we may substitute for grains. When you think of grains, think of breads, rice, cereals and pasta. Examples of root vegetables include white potatoes and the squash family, which includes sweet potatoes. People who have allergies and congestion should avoid eating white potatoes since they are a mucous forming food. Sweet potatoes are a better substitute since they are in an entirely different family of plants and do not generate mucous.

NOTE:
Food combining means that you eat fruits alone and either legumes with vegetables or grains with vegetables.

This is a simplified version of all of the food groups humans need for healthy nutrition. As you progress even further into the vegan concept, this diagram will help you learn how these foods interrelate in what is called "food combining." In essence, this means you eat fruits alone, and either legumes with vegetables <u>or</u> grains with vegetables. Food combining is aimed at optimizing digestion to create the most energy efficient metabolism you can achieve.

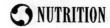

Is There Enough Protein in a Vegan Diet?

The first question people instinctively ask when I talk about a vegan diet is, "How do you get enough protein?" In fact, we are continually sold on the idea that we need dense protein foods, such as meat, poultry, fish and dairy products, in order to get adequate protein. Consequently, Americans consume approximately 18-20% protein in their diets. Is this really healthy?

NOTE:
. . . Americans consume approximately 18-20% protein in their diets. Is this really healthy?

Our Protein Requirements

Let's determine the protein requirements for "the new" Boris who now weighs 180 pounds and, with his walking, is in the moderately active group. Therefore, he requires 2,580 Calories per day. Wow! Even though Boris lost 20 pounds, he can enjoy eating nearly as many Calories as he did before . . . because of his activity!

First, let's calculate his absolute minimum protein requirement. When doing this arithmetic, it's easy for lay people to get lost in the unfamiliar units of the metric system. Therefore, I've converted grams, grams/day and grams/kilogram into the more simple to understand units of Calories per day and % protein in your diet. These results are recorded in Table 3.3.

If we did not nourish ourselves with proteins, to make up for it, our bodies would breakdown approximately 25 grams of its own protein each day.[30] After making the calculations, we can then say that, at the <u>very</u> <u>minimum</u>, Boris needs 100 Calories of protein per day, or 3.9% of his calories from protein.

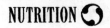

However, the <u>Recommended</u> <u>Daily</u> <u>Allowance</u> (RDA) for Americans is 0.8 grams of protein per kilogram of body weight.[31] According to this recommendation, Boris needs 262 protein Calories per day or 10% protein . . . more than three times the absolute minimum requirement. The RDA gives a liberal allowance to compensate for the "efficiency of utilization, which is typical of the mixed protein in the average American diet."[32] Now, compare this to the amount of protein <u>consumed</u> in the average American diet of 18-20%, Table 3.4.

Table 3.4
THE DAILY PROTEIN REQUIREMENTS FOR "THE NEW" BORIS
A Moderately Active 180 Pound Person Who Requires
2,580 Calories per Day

	Protein Calories per day	% Calories from Protein
Absoulute Minimum Requirement	100	3.9%
RDA of Protein	262	10%
Average Daily Diet		18-20%

NOTE:
. . . instead of worrying about how to get <u>enough</u> protein, should be worrying about how to avoid getting <u>too</u> <u>much</u> protein!

I am emphasizing the issue of our excessive protein consumption to help dispel the myth that we need dense protein foods like meat and dairy products to maintain optimal health. Vegan nutrition provides more than enough protein for total well being. To be sure, higher protein intake is required in athletes, pregnant women, convalescing adults and people with some diseases. However, the average healthy adult, instead of worrying about how to get <u>enough</u> protein, should be worrying about how to avoid getting <u>too</u> <u>much</u> protein!

What About "Essential" Amino Acids?

People often ask if vegetarian foods contain all of the essential amino acids . . . those building blocks of protein that the body does not manufacture on its own. The common misconception is that vegetarian diets are bad for you because either they don't provide enough protein or enough of the essential amino acids. Compare the essential amino acids contained in legumes (lentils and soy), vegetables (sunflower sprouts), human milk and meat in Table 3.5. Clearly, two out of the four food groups of vegetarian foods contain more than adequate concentrations of the essential amino acids, as well as the percentage of protein you need.

Table 3.5
ESSENTIAL AMINO ACIDS IN VARIOUS FOODS*

Essential Amino Acids	Lentils	Soy	Sunflower Sprouts	Human Milk	Meat
Tryptophan	0.22	0.53	0.06	0.10	0.22
Threonine	0.90	1.50	0.15	0.28	0.83
Isoleusine	1.32	2.05	0.21	0.34	0.98
Leucine	1.76	2.95	0.30	0.57	1.54
Lysine	1.53	2.41	0.12	0.41	1.64
Methionine	0.18	0.51	0.07	0.13	0.47
Phenyalanine	1.10	1.90	0.20	0.27	0.77
Valine	1.36	2.01	0.21	0.39	1.04
Arginine	1.91	2.76	0.30	0.25	1.21
Histidine	0.55	0.91	0.09	0.14	0.65
Total Protein	25%	35%	4%	1.4%	19%

*From: Kulvinskas, V. **Sprout for the Love of Everybody.** 21st Century Publications, Fairfield, IA. Rounded off to the nearest one hundredth.

Furthermore, it has been found that vegetarians do not need to mix certain foods together at each meal, such as combining beans with rice, in order to get a "complete protein." Not only are vegan foods complete in and of themselves, but if essential amino acids are not taken in at one meal, they may be eaten at subsequent meals without producing any protein deficiency.[33]

Making It Work

Usually, when people consider moving from diets on the left of the Nutrition Spectrum into vegetarianism, they think they will find the food tasteless, boring and unfulfilling. There's nothing further from the truth, especially as you allow your body to cleanse and detoxify. Vegetarian foods provide a vibrant mixture of colors, tastes and textures . . . a wide assortment of spices herbs and flavors . . . and a variety of dishes, snacks and desserts. Indeed, the whole lifestyle change associated with vegan nutrition is an exciting experience and the best part is that you will create a whole new sense of well being.

I've included some very useful information in the practical applications section at the end of this chapter. Also, there are a number of excellent books in the resources section to help you get started on the vegetarian way (9,10,11). As you wean away from the heavy rich foods that drag you down and create unwellness, you'll likely dedicate yourself more and more to total living foods such as you will find in the Natural Hygiene Nutrition Diet.

The Natural Hygiene Diet

The absolute optimal nutrition, one enjoyed by hundreds of thousands of Americans, is the natural hygiene diet (12,13). This nutrition is based upon the vegan concept but utilizes only fresh or raw foods. In addition, most natural hygienists practice proper food combining, which I discussed in describing the four food groups above.

The Living Foods Program

A special sub-classification of natural hygiene nutrition is called the Living Foods Program. This emphasizes enzyme-rich sprouted seeds and grains, as well as fermented foods. This concept is particularly therapeutic for individuals in the unwell population and may even be helpful for those who suffer from disease, especially when orthodox medicine fails.

NOTE:
We truly are what we eat.

The most important risk factor we have for any disease condition is our genetics. In addition to that, however, is the risk factor involving what we eat. We truly are what we eat. As Hippocrates said, "Let your food be your medicine, and your medicine be your food." One of the best centers in the country that trains people in the living foods life style is the Hippocrates Health Institute in West Palm Beach, Florida (14).

Reasons Why The Natural Hygiene Concept Is Optimal

Freshly prepared, live vegetarian foods are easily less than 10% fat and, therefore, minimize the diseases associated with a high fat, low fiber diet. Furthermore, these foods do not contain the animal fats that cause inflammation. Because of their low fat content, we ingest far fewer oil soluble poisons and toxins when eating them, especially if the foods are organically grown. Typically, vegetarian diets contain a much healthier combination of the three foods; carbohydrates, 80%; proteins, 10%; and fats, 10%. In addition, the carbohydrates in these foods, being in their natural state, are complex. Therefore, we do not suffer from the many causes of refined sugars, such as hypoglycemia and candidiasis, a condition caused by yeast overgrowth in our bodies. Moreover, the protein load is kept at a reasonable level to maintain a healthier acid base balance in our bodies.

All of these reasons alone would suffice to support Natural Hygiene as the optimal in nutrition, but there is one other consideration which happens to coincide with the most exciting movement in today's nutrition.

Supplements

Nutritional supplementation, or taking vitamins and minerals, has grabbed the headlines in America. Perhaps there is justification for the use of supplements, since the additives in our food and the heavily refined processing of the Standard American Diet have left us with an unhealthy, obese population. The justification for taking supplements is based upon a re-discovered hypothesis explaining tissue destruction and the cause of disease and aging known as the free radical hypothesis.

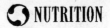

Free Radicals

Free radicals are constantly being formed throughout our bodies during the normal course of oxidative metabolism as well as from a host of physiological stresses. These stresses include environmental radiation and pollution; toxins in our food chain, as well as those produced in our colons (see page 141); and drugs and tissue ischemia from atherosclerosis (see page 13). The basic element of matter, from our tissues, down to our cells and molecules, is composed of atoms which normally are surrounded by paired electrons. Free radicals are formed when atoms lose one electron leaving an unpaired electron in its orbit, Figure 3.5.

Thousands of these free radicals scurry throughout our bodies like Pac men searching for and robbing electrons from the atoms of healthy cells. One target includes the membranes of our cells. The loss of electrons from cell membranes distorts these cells leading to tissue damage and chronic degenerative disease such as atherosclerosis. A second favorite target of free radicals is the DNA molecule which, when robbed of its electrons, leads to the death of the cell or the abnormal proliferation of these cells which is, in effect, cancer.

NOTE:
. . . free radicals scurry throughout our body like Pac men searching for and robbing electrons from the atoms of healthy cells.

Antioxidants

Fortunately, vitamins, for example from fruits and vegetables, contribute their electrons to the free radicals resulting in "healthy atoms" at the sacrifice of the vitamins, Figure 3.5. Since oxygen is involved at the chemical level in the formation of free radicals, these vitamins are called "antioxidants." The primary antioxidant vitamins include beta carotene (a pre-cursor to vitamin A), vitamin C and vitamin E. Numerous scientific studies have shown that the antioxidant properties of these vitamins stabilize the walls of our arteries and prevent atherosclerosis.[34] In addition, currently available data are compatible with the possibility that antioxidant vitamins may decrease the risk of cancer.[35] Unfortunately, the highly refined, processed foods of our Standard American Diet have been depleted of these antioxidants.

This has created a burgeoning industry selling antioxidants. Most of the companies claim a special mixture or patented formula that has "proven effective," especially with testimonials from sponsoring athletes and other entertainers. Because there is such a variety of pills, I have listed the contents of a generic formula for those of you who choose this approach, Table 3.6.

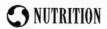

Figure 3.5
FREE RADICALS AND THEIR DAMAGE TO HEALTHY TISSUE

VITAMINS FROM FRUITS, VEGETABLES, NUTS AND BEANS

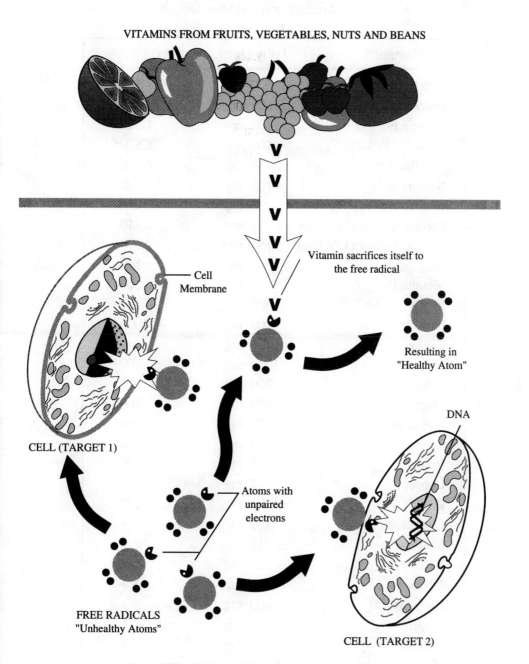

Vitamin sacrifices itself to the free radical

Cell Membrane

Resulting in "Healthy Atom"

DNA

CELL (TARGET 1)

Atoms with unpaired electrons

FREE RADICALS "Unhealthy Atoms"

CELL (TARGET 2)

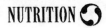

Table 3.6
GENERIC FORMULA FOR A DAILY MULTI-VITAMIN
with AntiOxidants and Minerals

Vitamin	Daily Dose*		% US RDA
Beta Carotene (Vit A)	25,000	iu	500
Ascorbic Acid (Vit C)	1,200	mg	2,000
Vitamin E	400	iu	1,330
Thiamine (Vit B_1)	100	mg	6,670
Riboflavin (Vit B_2)	75	mg	4,410
Niacin (Vit B_3)	105	mg	520
Niacinamide (Vit B_3)	30	mg	600
Pyridoxine (Vit B_6)	75	mg	3,750
Cyanocobalamin (Vit B_{12})	150	mcg	2,500
Folic Acid	400	mcg	100
Vitamin D	800	iu	200
Biotin	300	mcg	100
Pantothence	100	mg	1000
Choline	100	mg	+
Calcium	1000	mg	100
Phosphorus	300	mg	30
Magnesium	400	mg	100
Potassium	50	mg	+
Iodine	225	mcg	150
Iron	15	mg	80
Copper	2	mg	100
Zinc	15	mg	100
Chromium	100	mcg	+
Manganese	15	mcg	+
Bataine HCl	37	mg	+
Bentonite	100	mg	+
Bioflavinoids	100	mg	+
Inositol	75	mg	+
PABA	75	mg	+

* Take in divided doses to avoid urinary excretion.

\+ No US RDA has been established.

By providing this formula, I am not sanctioning the use of pills in place of making fundamental changes in your nutritional lifestyle. Indeed, I question the approach that says, go ahead with your lifestyle that causes disease, we'll intervene with a pill . . . a quick fix. In fact, how were these pills formulated? What are they made of? This brings me to a fascinating question about vitamins.

Tomorrow's Supplement

How many vitamins were there ten years ago . . . how many are there today . . . and how many will there be in five to ten years? The answer, of course, depends upon the source of information and the definition of what a "vitamin" is. However, I suspect you're getting the point. Many new vitamins are certain to be discovered in the future. Where do these vitamins come from? Not just food, but fruits and vegetables!

NOTE:
. . . simply taking vitamins is not as nutritious as eating whole fruits and vegetables.

Let's explore this concept further. A dozen studies have shown that vegetarian diets are associated with a statistically significant decrease in incidence of colon cancer.[36] This is, presumably, due to their high content of antioxidant vitamins. Yet, when people are given antioxidant vitamins in pill form, there is no effect on the rate of colon polyps that lead to colon cancer.[37] One plausible explanation for the discrepancy between the benefits of whole food versus vitamin supplementation is that "dietary levels of antioxidant vitamins simply reflect the consumption of fruits and vegetables which, in turn, contain other substances that reduce the risk of colorectal cancer."[38] In other words, simply taking vitamins is not as nutritious as eating whole fruits and vegetables. There are dozens of micronutrients that have yet to be discovered from living foods.

The pills that manufacturers make are either synthesized or extracted vitamins, mainly from plants. If that's the case, doesn't it stand to reason that if we want the ultimate in nutrition . . . if we want today what will be identified as an essential "vitamin" tomorrow, we should nourish ourselves with their primal source . . . fresh vegetarian foods!

This brings me to a fascinating closure to the topic of supplements.

Phytochemicals

One of the newest and most exciting breakthroughs in modern nutrition is Phytochemicals (Phytos: Gr. = plant). There are hundreds of natural chemicals being extracted from fruits and vegetables that prevent diseases, particularly cancer.[39] Interestingly, these include plants that have been used in healing for centuries, such as the curciferous family (broccoli, cauliflower, brussel sprouts and turnips), cabbage (sauerkraut), soybeans and olives. Did your mother, like mine, ever tell you to eat lots of whole fruits and vegetables? It seems the older I get, the smarter she becomes! Even the National Council on Nutrition recommends including five daily servings of fruits and vegetables in our diets.

These phytochemicals protect us by a variety of mechanisms. For example, sulforaphanes from the broccoli family decrease breast cancer in laboratory animals. These phytochemicals activate intracellular enzymes that produce molecules which transport and dispose of invading carcinogenic toxins that we ingest or inhale. Phytochemicals from tomatoes, called p-coumaric and chlorogenic acid, block the synthesis of cancer-forming molecules. Cabbage contains phytochemicals that use up our endogenous enzymes which, otherwise, convert toxins into fragments that bind to DNA causing abnormal cell growth, or cancer.

Of course, the way to prevent disease such as cancer, is to avoid toxins in the first place. We do this by cutting out fat in our diets which carries with it excessive oil soluble toxins, as I discussed earlier. We stop smoking, avoid secondary smoke inhalation and help decrease air pollutants in our environment. We eat organic foods, free from toxic chemicals. Then, we practice optimal nutrition to protect our bodies from naturally occurring toxins, carcinogenic chemicals and free radicals by eating live whole fruits and vegetables. Indeed, optimal nutrition lies toward the right on the Nutrition Spectrum!

NOTE: *. . . optimal nutrition lies toward the right on the Nutrition Spectrum!*

Summary

Unknowingly, most Americans buy illness and disease. The Standard American diet is high in animal fat, deficient in fiber, highly refined and contains toxic chemicals. Yet, the food industry is simply practicing sound American economics selling what they perceive the customer wants . . . taste, convenience and cost. Unfortunately, this ignores the essential reason that we eat . . . health. We pay the price!

There is an epidemic in America called obesity. People become ill and develop disease. There is a fire sale in America called diets. People lose weight . . . put it back on . . . lose weight . . . and continue to yo yo! Weight management does not equate to changing your diet. Weight management does equate to changing your lifestyle. Fortunately, consumer awareness regarding food is on the rise, and the medical community is turning its attention to prevention through improved nutrition. We have the power to step toward optimal nutrition and, as we do, the food industry will surely follow.

Based upon where you are on the Nutrition Spectrum, begin improving your nutrition with smaller portions of meat, then emphasize fish and fowl or move into the lacto-vegetarian diet. These are all steps in the right direction. Then, consider decreasing dairy products even further since milk products contain excessive animal fat, dense protein and toxic chemicals and additives. Consider moving even further into optimal nutrition.

Indeed, humans are physiologically and anatomically herbivores. Optimal nutrition for us is the Vegan diet. This is particularly true of organically grown, fresh, living fruits and vegetables. Complete vegetarian nutrition provides all of the essential amino acids, enough protein, the essential fatty acids and all of the health promoting micronutrients we need . . . plus some.

Medical science shows that vegetarian populations have a decreased incidence of heart disease and cancer. Yet, vitamins alone are not complete replacements. Whole living fruits and vegetables contain chemicals (phytochemicals) that combat disease and promote health.

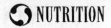

Practical Applications

The following are basic concepts and hints that will help you make a transition from high fat, low fiber, highly refined foods to a healthier nutrition as you move toward the right along the Nutrition Spectrum.

This is not a race. Make the transition work for <u>you</u>. Whether that translates into "all or nothing" or taking it one step at a time, begin <u>now</u>! Get the help of your significant other, family and friends. Surround yourself with lots of reading materials and recipes. Locate and visit your nearest health food store for the items discussed here. In case there is no health food store in your area, I've included instructions, resource books, recipes and companies where you can order everything you will need to get started. Experiment, explore and have fun!

Supplies and Equipment

Most well stocked kitchens contain the necessary utensils, pots and pans and other equipment needed for vegan recipes. Get out your high speed blender, steamer, wok, toaster and food processor. Obtain some quart glass jars, gauze or fine meshed screen and thick rubber bands to experiment with sprouting. Buy a high quality juicer. I personally use and recommend the Champion Juicer which is one of the most versatile, yet reasonably priced, machines available (15).

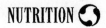

Protein Alternatives

Throughout this chapter I have emphasized that the concentrated sources of protein we ingest in the form of meat and dairy products carry with them a number of risks to our health. They are high in fat and low in fiber, contain toxins from their food chains and contribute to excessive protein that acidifies our systems. Fortunately, there are many protein alternatives that are both nutritious and delicious.

TOFU is the most versatile, high protein, low fat vegetable-protein food available. It's made from pressed soybean curd and, owing to its neutral taste, absorbs flavors from all the foods with which it is combined. Tofu can be prepared in a variety of ways, such as, mashed, braised, baked, steamed or grilled. It's a marvelous substitute for meat, eggs or cheese. It comes vacuum packed in water so, after you open the package, store it in a closed lid container under water and frequently rinse it.

TEMPEH is an excellent meat substitute with less fat than tofu and the consistency of "hamburger." It is made from pressed fermented soybeans plus other grains, and it is high in vitamin B_{12}. Due to its consistency, it can be used to make vegeburgers, kabobs, stews, barbecues or stirfrys.

SPROUTS are a <u>superb</u> food source for a number of reasons. They have high concentrations of easily digestible proteins, living enzymes, minimally complex sugars and essential fatty acids. Most seeds, grains and legumes can be sprouted. With a little practice, you can easily apply the following instructions to grow the sprouts that best serve your needs.

Wash about a half cup of seeds or grains to remove debris and then soak them in a large glass jar overnight to get rid of growth inhibiting enzymes. Cover the jar with gauze or screening secured with thick rubber bands and drain off the water. Rinse thoroughly, drain completely and keep them in the dark for one to two days to initiate the sprouting process. On day three, put them in direct sunlight to generate chlorophyll if the leaves are green, such as in sunflower sprouts. If the sprouts do not turn green, such as garbanzo and mungbeans sprouts, continue to sprout them in the dark. Throughout this process, rinse them every eight to twelve hours and keep them in a cool environment to minimize growth of mold. After three to five days, use the sprouts in salads and sandwiches and add them to vegetable juices.

You may obtain seeds and grains from your local health food store. In addition, I encourage you to obtain the informative catalog from the mail-order house, Seeds of Change (16).

TAHINI is made from ground, unsalted sesame seeds. It contains 35% protein, is rich in calcium and phosphorous, but has a high fat content. Tahini is an excellent addition to recipes for hummus, dressings and sauces. Use only raw, organic tahini.

SPIRULINA and OTHER ALGAES could be considered the essence of life since they are at the bottom of our food chain. Algae has characteristics of bacteria (no nucleus), plants (contains chlorophyll) and animals (its cell wall is a plasma membrane lacking cellulose). It has concentrated, easily digestible protein; carbohydrates; an essential omega 6 fatty acid, gamma linolenic acid; beta carotene, a precursor to vitamin A; vitamins B and E; iron; and chlorophyll. Since algae is a natural unprocessed food, it contains other antioxidants and "vitamins" that we

NOTE:
If you can't eat whole vegetarian foods . . . algae is an excellent supplement.

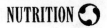

haven't discovered yet. Alone, algae has a slightly musty taste, but it can be made into a tasty drink, since it takes on the flavor of any fruit or vegetable juice with which it is mixed. It can also be taken in capsule form.

Algae products can be obtained at health food stores or multilevel marketing companies such as Cell Tech (17) and Light Force (18).

Dairy Alternatives

NOTE:
. . . you can make up to forty delicious, dairy free milks .

GRAIN MILKS are creamy, sweet and a perfect alternative to animal milk. They are produced from either brown rice, soybeans or a combination of both. There are a host of different milks on the market with a variety of flavors such as plain, vanilla, carob (chocolate) and various fruits. Some milks are produced with a low fat content or fortified with protein, vitamins and minerals. Thanks to our health-conscious public, they are now available on the shelves of many regular grocery stores.

Rice milk, for example Rice Dream, is made from brown rice which is the most easily digested and least allergenic of all the grains. Soy milk is produced by a number of different companies such as Eden Soy, Soy Moo, Vita Soy and Westbrae. Amazake is a combination of rice and soy milk and contains beneficial micro-flora.

In addition to milk, most of these products are also made into delicious natural ice creams.

NUT and SEED MILKS are other excellent dairy milk replacements and can easily be prepared at home. They contain a concentrated source of protein, essential fatty acids, vitamins A, B, D, and E, calcium, phosphorous, potassium, magnesium, iron and other trace minerals. With a variety of nuts,

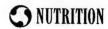

sweeteners, spices and other natural additives, there are recipes with which you can make up to forty delicious, dairy free milks (19). Just to get you started, try almond nut or sesame seed milk by following these simple directions:

1. Soak 1 cup of organic raw almonds <u>or</u> sesame seeds over night.
2. Discard the water and rinse.
3. Place the nuts or seeds in a blender and add one tablespoon of maple syrup or another one of the sweeteners discussed below. Blend with approximately two to three cups water. Add more or less water to create the creamy consistency you desire.
4. Strain through a fine mesh strainer and refrigerate.

Enjoy the milk as a delicious nutritious drink, poured over cereal or combined in food preparations.

Breads and Cereals

There are three concerns that many people have with the breads we commonly purchase in grocery stores: 1) their use of processed refined grains, 2) their excessive reliance on wheat and 3) the presence of yeast. Most people are aware that using whole grain bread is more nutritious than processed grains. The refining process destroys the germ which contains the essential nutrients and gets rid of the chafe which adds fiber. Even enriched or fortified refined breads, lacking the germ and chafe of the grain, do not compare in nutritive value to whole grain bread.

NOTE:
Even enriched or fortified refined breads . . . do not compare in nutritive value to whole grain bread.

Many food allergists claim that the three offending food groups in our society include meats, dairy products and wheat. Wheat is everywhere in our food supply.

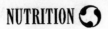

Fortunately, there are a variety of diverse grain alternatives in addition to the other commonly used grains, rice, rye and oats. These grains do not produce the allergic reactions associated with wheat, and they do not contain gluten, which causes intestinal problems in many people. All of these grains can be cooked whole as a food, sprouted or obtained as cereal flakes and flour to make breads.

Wheat Alternatives

AMARANTH is an ancient, Central American grain common to the once thriving civilizations like the Aztecs and Mayans. It's a tiny, creamy, beige-colored seed with a nutty flavor.

BUCKWHEAT is a triangular shaped grain (groats) related to the rhubarb family. Hulled, toasted buckwheat groats, called Kasha, yield a distinctive earthy flavor. Sprouted buckwheat provides a leafy sprout good for juicing with vegetable drinks.

KAMUT is an ancient Egyptian grain related to the common ancestors of wheat. It's higher in protein and other essential minerals and produces less sensitivity than hybridized wheat.

QUINOA is an ancient South American grain associated with the Inca civilization who called it the "mother grain." It is considered the best source of vegetable protein, due to its outstanding balance of essential amino acids. If you purchase it raw, thoroughly wash it to remove the bitter saponins contained in the grain's coat that act as a natural pest deterrent.

MILLET is a tiny, round yellow grain with a nutty flavor and fluffy texture. It is a versatile grain and can be eaten cooked or toasted.

SPELT, like Kamut, is a non-hybrid wheat. It is closer to wheat in taste and character than any other grain, but is better tolerated by people who are sensitive to wheat. Spelt bread and cereal provide an excellent alternative to wheat.

TEFF is the tiniest of all grains. It has the highest fiber content of any grain and is particularly good in combination with other grains.

Yeast Alternatives

Some people, especially those diagnosed with candidiasis, prefer breads that have been prepared without yeast. Alternatives include sprouted, unleavened and sourdough breads. Look for these breads in the refrigerated section of a health food store.

SPROUTED BREAD (Essene, Manna) consists of whole sprouts compounded together into loafs. They are delicious when thinly sliced, toasted and lightly covered with a natural vegetarian oil spread.

UNLEAVENED rye bread is prepared in compacted loaves without yeast and commonly contains other seeds such as sunflower or sesame.

SOURDOUGH bread is made to rise with a special fermented culture and, therefore, does not contain yeast. A variety of different grains are used.

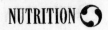

Sweeteners

Highly refined processed sugar is void of any other nutrients and is a concentrated from of simple sugar, which can trigger dramatic swings in metabolism. These metabolic swings may produce high blood sugar (hyperglycemia), low blood sugar (hypoglycemia) or a multitude of symptoms, such as palpitations, light headedness, sweating, blurred vision and headaches. Unfortunately, the commonly used artificial sweeteners are often associated with allergies or symptoms such as headaches, dizziness and fatigue.

Fortunately, there are a number of <u>natural</u> sweeteners. Many of these are foods that are metabolized more slowly and, thus, do not create rapid swings in our blood sugar.

BARELY MALT is derived from organic, sprouted barley grain, contains complex sugars, and can be obtained in a syrup or powder. The amber colored syrup is stronger in flavor than honey and milder than molasses. It is 50-70% as sweet as sugar. On the other hand, the powder has a sweetness 20 times that of sugar. There are approximately three calories in a dash, which substitutes for two teaspoons of sugar. Bronner's barley malt powder is a specially blended natural sweetener consisting of fruit juice solids, minerals, spices and herbs.

BROWN RICE SYRUP is made from organic brown rice, which is cooked and treated with natural enzymes that produce nutritious complex sugars. It resembles honey but is of natural vegetarian origin and not as sweet.

CAROB POWDER is derived from the seed pod of an evergreen tree. Although it is not really a sweetener substitute, it is an excellent replacement for chocolate. Carob is mainly a carbohydrate and has some minerals and B vitamins, but no caffeine or fats. Look for raw, untoasted carob.

DATE SUGAR is made from dried, crushed dates and provides a granulated sweetener similar to raw sugar that can be sprinkled on foods or dissolved in the preparation of foods.

DRIED FRUITS soaked in water overnight provide a "sweetened" water that can be used in preparing nut milks and other foods. Avoid eating dried fruit alone, since it is extremely high in fruit sugar (fructose) and causes reactions similar to refined white sugar.

MAPLE SYRUP is the most natural sugar substitute, so long as it is authentic and without preservatives or other additives. It has little other nutritional value and does contain simple sugars, so use it sparingly.

STEVIA REBAUDIANA is an herb derived from a shrub and when processed into a concentrated form has a sweetness 30 to 80 times that of sugar. It has a licorice-like taste, and because it has no calories or fat, it is particularly useful for people who have diabetes, hypoglycemia or candidiasis. Note, however, that the FDA has banned Stevia as a sugar substitute. Therefore, use it at your own risk. It can be obtained in prepackaged dropper bottles from Sunrider International who sell it as a skin care preparation called, Suncare (20).

Oils

NOTE:

Envision which you would rather have floating around in your blood and joints, liquid oil or congealed lard.

Plant oils are more nutritious than animal fats since they have less risk for promoting atherosclerosis. Plants contain essential oils, which are fatty acids that our bodies cannot synthesize. There are two categories of these fatty acids called omega 3 (linolenic acids) and omega 6 (linoleic acids). These oils are liquid at room and even cold temperatures; as opposed to saturated animal fatty acids which congeal even at room temperatures; for example, bacon fat. Envision which you would rather have floating around in your blood and joints, liquid oil or congealed lard.

Hydrogenated margarines are re-configured plant oils that make them spreadable at room temperature. It turns out, however, that their rearranged molecular configuration is harmful to the cells of our bodies. Non-hydrogenated canola oil spread is a healthy natural vegetable oil substitute. Butter, in small amounts, is healthier than hydrogenated margarine but low in essential fatty acids. Keep in mind that even "good" plant oils have the same number of calories as any fat.

Buy oils in small quantities and keep them refrigerated in dark bottles. Look for virgin cold pressed oils which have not been heated. Avoid heating any oil, since it creates cancer producing chemicals (carcinogens). It is preferable to add oils to food after the food is cooked. Use water or vegetable broth for "steam-sauteed" food. Arrowhead Mills, Omega Nutrition and Jaffe Brothers provide certified oils which are properly prepared and packaged (21,22,23).

CANOLA OIL is one of the most nutritious and balanced oils. It contains the essential fatty acids and is rich in vitamins E and K, chlorophyll and beta carotene. Canola oil spread, congealed with xanthum and guara gums, makes a healthy substitute for hydrogenated margarine. Look for a brand labeled, Spectrum.

FLAXSEED OIL is undoubtedly the <u>most</u> <u>nutritious</u> <u>oil</u> available, because it contains both of the essential omega 3 and omega 6 fatty acid groups. In addition, it contains beta carotene, vitamin E and lignans, which are special nutrients beneficial in preventing disease. Flaxseed oil is not found on grocery store shelves because of a restricted shelf life. You can find it in the refrigerated section of health food stores or purchase it from the sources listed above. Use it for salad dressings or in prepared foods that do not have to be heated. Of all the oils, flaxseed is the best for anyone with essential fatty acid deficiency, and it can be taken in the oil form or in capsules.

OLIVE OIL has a rich, aromatic flavor and is the most commonly used all around oil. It contains monounsaturated fatty acids, but little of the omega 3 and 6 varieties. It can be used for light sauteing, baking or making salad dressings, sauces and spreads. Caruthers is an excellent brand.

SAFFLOWER OIL is a versatile vegetable oil rich in polyunsaturated fatty acids, especially the omega 6's. It can be used for light sauteing, baking, salad dressing, sauces and dips.

NAYONAISE is an excellent substitute for mayonnaise. It's made from all natural vegetable ingredients, low in fat and sodium, and it's cholesterol free. It has a soybean base with canola oil, spices and vegetable gums to make it a rich, tangy tasting spread.

NOTE:
FLAXSEED OIL is undoubtedly the <u>*most*</u> <u>*nutritious*</u> <u>*oil*</u> *available...*

Salt Substitutes and Other Condiments

The amount of salt (sodium chloride) we consume in our diets is dangerously high. The average daily intake is in excess of five grams, yet we need less than half that amount for normal physiological function. Excessive salt intake holds water in our bodies that causes tissue swelling and affects our kidneys leading to high blood pressure. Simply exchanging other minerals, such as magnesium for sodium, decreases blood pressure in some hypertensive patients without having to rely on any medication.[40]

In addition, the exclusive use of sodium chloride deprives us of other essential trace minerals. Fortunately, we can add these minerals to our diets by using sea salts from natural sea vegetables or from soybean extracts.

KELP POWDER is a complete sea based mineral that can be sprinkled on food just like regular salt.

DULSE is a mild tasting, purple sea vegetable that can be eaten dried or used after soaking in sauces or soups. It is high in protein and rich in iodine, iron and other minerals.

NORI consists of crispy thin sheets of pressed sea vegetables that contain B vitamins and minerals. It is used to roll around chopped vegetables, cooked grains and nut patties to make Sushi rolls.

OTHER SEA VEGETABLES include Arame, Kombu, Hijike and Wakame.

BRAGG LIQUID AMINO ACIDS is made from soy beans and water and could be considered a salty, liquid vegetable protein. It is widely used as a flavoring and salt substitute in vegetarian cuisine but is high in sodium and, therefore, should be diluted 50/50 with water. It has a delicious flavor and is used in dressings, sauces, gravies and soups. Braggs' can be used to sauté in place of oil. In addition, you can put some in a spray bottle for flavoring popcorn.

SOY SAUCE and TAMARI are made from fermented soy beans, water, grains and sea salts. They are excellent spices and are used in sauces, soups and in the preparation of foods. However, you need to be aware that they are high in salt content. For example, 1 tablespoon of Tamari equals your normal daily intake of sodium.

MISO is made from aged, fermented soy beans and either brown rice, barley or garbanzo beans. It is high in protein, the B vitamins, enzymes and friendly bacteria. Miso is used in sauces, soups and main dishes, or it may be used as a dressing in and of itself.

NUTRITIONAL YEAST is packaged as flakes and has no activity to raise bread. It is high in vitamin B complex, including vitamin B_{12}. Although not salty, it is an excellent salt replacement and has a gentle, distinctive flavor when sprinkled on steamed vegetables, salads or popcorn.

A Few Snacks and a Quick Breakfast

AIR POPPED POPCORN is delicious when garnished with drops of olive or flaxseed oil, sprayed with Braggs' and granulated with non-nutritional yeast.

HUMMUS is wonderful on low-fat, baked tortilla chips, pita bread or "veggie sticks." One recipe for hummus is as follows:

> Mix the following ingredients in a blender or food processor:
> 1 can (15 oz) boiled garbanzo beans
> 3 tablespoons tamari
> 1-2 cloves of garlic
> 2 tablespoons lemon juice
> Dash of cumin
> 2 tablespoons minced onion
> Add water to reach desired consistency

After blending, sprinkle with parsley or cayenne pepper.

GUACAMOLE DIP is great with low fat tortilla chips, pita bread or "veggie sticks."

> To prepare, blend the following ingredients:
> 2-3 mashed avocados
> 1 small, diced red bell pepper
> 1 tablespoon kelp
> 1/2 chopped onion
> 1/4 teaspoon cayenne pepper (to taste)
> Juice from 1 lemon
> 1 clove crushed garlic
> 2 tablespoons Nayonaise

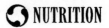

MUNCHIES

Food	% Cal as FAT
Pretzels, unsalted	8
Air popped popcorn	9
Baked tortilla chips	9
Baked potato chips	9
Rice cakes or chips	15

A QUICK NUTRITIOUS BREAKFAST (serving size, 1 person)

1. Soak the following in water overnight in separate bowls:
     1 cup of stone ground oats
     1/2 cup raw organic almonds
     1/2 cup organic raisins

2. Pour off and discard the water from the oats and almonds.

3. Place the almonds in a blender, pour the sweetened water from the raisins into the blender and blend.

4. Strain the almond milk through a strainer.

5. Mix the raisins, oats and sweetened almond milk in a bowl for a delicious and nutritious granola-like cereal.

BANANA "ICE CREAM" WITH "CHOCOLATE" SAUCE

1. Prepare carob "chocolate" sauce as follows:
     1 cup carob powder
     2 tablespoons date sugar (or sweeten to taste)
     Stir in water and slowly heat to a thick hot fudge sauce consistency

2. Freeze peeled ripe bananas in a freezer in Ziploc baggies.

3. Homogenize in a blender or Champion juicer.

4. Pour the chocolate sauce over the banana "ice cream."

Wow!

VEGETABLE JUICE

NOTE:

I recommend drinking one frresh vegetable juice a day to boost your daily nutrition.

Any fresh vegetables in combination or alone (such as carrot juice) are an excellent source of protein, carbohydrates, minerals, vitamins and other essential nutrients. Wash the vegetables with a stiff brush and rinse well. Juice in a juicer or, if you don't have one, a regular blender, in which case you will need to strain the juice.

A basic vegetable juice combination can be made as follows:
1 bunch of celery
1 cucumber
1 cup of fresh sprouts such as sunflower or buckwheat,
1 clove garlic or a small cut of ginger

I recommend drinking one fresh vegetable juice a day to boost your daily nutrition.

These are just a few recipes to get you started. I encourage you to obtain some of the excellent recipe books that apply to various locations along the right of the Nutritional Spectrum (24,25,26,27).

Resources

I want to encourage you again to move along the Nutrition Spectrum at your own pace. For example, gradually wean yourself off the heavy, fat laden foods that cause cravings and sluggish after effects. Retrain your tastebuds and allow your physiological and biochemical systems to accommodate to a lighter and healthier diet. For those of you who are ready to change, perhaps because of disease or you just plain don't feel well, take bigger steps and remember, a few steps forward with occasional back stepping still gets you where your want to go. As I have mentioned throughout this chapter, there are excellent resources that can help us along this path toward optimal nutrition.

Marc Sorenson, Ed.D has written a very good book for lay people entitled, **MegaHealth**, in which he documents the unhealthy effects of high fat diets and the benefits of good nutrition and exercise (1). In addition, his National Institute of Fitness provides an excellent, cost effective retreat where people eat low fat SAD, AHA and vegetarian foods, combined with hiking in the foothills of Utah's Snow Canyon State Park. I especially recommend this for hesitant people who are making their first transition into better nutrition and exercise.

The Pritikin concept offers a good transition through the SAD/AHA nutrition into a 20% fat diet. It allows lean meats, fish, fowl and dairy products. This diet is especially easy to follow since many food items are prepared to the Pritikin specifications and available in standard grocery stores and restaurants. In addition, there is a Pritikin Longevity Center in both Florida and California where excellent education and hands-on experience teaches the basic principles of this nutrition (3,4). I encourage patients to read the first section of his latest book, **The Pritikin Promise,** for

NOTE:
Retrain your tastebuds and allow your physiological and biochemical systems to accommodate to a lighter and healthier diet.

an introduction to the principles of low fat nutrition (4).

Dean Ornish, M.D., brought the value of alternative lifestyles to orthodox medicine. By utilizing accepted scientific techniques, he proved that proper nutrition, exercise and stress management can prevent heart disease and reverse atherosclerosis as well (5). His nutrition is based to the right, but within the lacto-vegetarian diet where he allows skim milk, low fat yogurt and egg whites. This would be a relatively easy jump to make for anyone who is serious about moving from the SAD fare into more optimal nutrition. Furthermore, his institute offers a one week program to learn and experience his program (6).

Neal D. Bernard, M.D. is president of the Physicians Committee for Responsible Medicine, a nationwide group of physicians who promote preventive medicine through healthier food choices (7). Dr. Bernard created the four basic food groups for vegetarian foods. You can learn more about eating well for better health and about the four food groups by reading his book, **The Power of Your Plate**, and contacting the Committee headquarters (8).

There are a number of excellent books to get you started in vegetarian nutrition. For starters, I recommend the **Vegetarian Starter Kit** available from the Committee for Responsible Medicine (9), or a comprehensive, yet simply written, book by Michael Klapper, M.D. called, **Vegan Nutrition** (10). The most complete resource is the **McDougall Plan** by John McDougall, M.D. and Mary McDougall (11).

For those who are suffering in the unwell population described in the Health Continuum or desire to incorporate a nutritional approach in treating disease, I recommend the Natural Hygiene and, more specifically, the Living Foods approach. In fact, Natural Hygiene is a staple diet for thousands of Americans who, as a result, enjoy excellent health. Further information can be obtained by contacting that organization and reading the book, **Fit for Life** (12,13). The Hippocrates Health Institute in West Palm Beach, Florida, stands at the pinnacle of optimal nutrition (14). The Director, Brian Clement, has updated and created a comprehensive program which brings the Living Foods concept to guests from all over the world. The Hippocrates Institute is particularly beneficial for those with compromised health or individuals interested in learning and experiencing the ultimate in nutrition and a healthy lifestyle.

The Champion juicer (15) is a masticating machine that breaks up the cells of fruits and vegetables giving you optimal amounts of fiber, enzymes, vitamins and minerals. With a simple adjustment, you can juice, grate or homogenize. This allows you to create fruit and vegetable juices, sherbet cocktail, grated vegetables, sorbet and ice cream substitutes, purees and sauces and nut butters.

Seeds of Change is a mail order company whose catalog will provide you with a new world of instructive information on all imaginable seeds and grains (16). They believe that biodiversity in our food system provides superior plant-based nutrition necessary for a healthy, peaceful world.

NOTE:
. . . biodiversity in our food system provides superior plant-based nutrition . . .

Cell Tech (17) and Light Force (18) are multilevel companies that distribute supplements derived from natural products, including algae.

Candia L. Cole wrote **Not Milk . . . Nutmilks,** consisting of 40 original dairy-free milk recipes (19). It's amazing how creamy, smooth, and sweet these nutritious milks are.

Stevia has been banned by the FDA as a sweetener substitute, however, you can obtain it as a herbal skincare preparation called Suncare from Sunrider International, a multilevel company (20).

The following are among the best most reliable mail order companies where you can purchase certified, organic foods including nuts, seeds, grains and oils: Arrowhead Mills (21), Omega Nutrition (22) and Jaffe Brothers (23).

NOTE:

There are a number of excellent recipe books that will help you as you move toward optimal nutrition.

There are a number of excellent recipe books that will help you as you move toward optimal nutrition. If you are still in the SAD or AHA diets, I encourage you to explore foods at the right of the lacto-vegetarian diet with Dr. Ornish's book, **Eat More, Weigh Less** (24). He teaches low fat nutrition using egg whites, skim milk and low fat yogurt with over 250 recipes. In addition, he emphasizes improving your health by healing emotional pain, loneliness and isolation in your life.

One of the best all around cookbooks for part-time vegetarians, fully committed vegetarians or anyone who is just trying to eat more healthfully is Marilyn Diamond's, **The American Vegetarian Cookbook** (25). In addition to over 500 full-menu recipes, her book is chock-full of extras such as nutrition charts, how to set up a vegan kitchen, a list of pantry items to get, a vegan shopping list, thirst quenchers and "fix-it-fast" recipes.

Moving further to the right along the Nutrition Spectrum, is an excellent recipe book by Rita Romano entitled, **Dining in the Raw, Cooking with the Buff** (26). Rita offers nutritional advice and sound cuisine to show how dining with high enzyme foods can increase your longevity and provide rejuvenating powers.

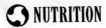

A definitive primer to the Hippocrates living foods concept is given by Steven Levine and Brenda Star in their book, **Living with Live Foods** (27). In addition to recipes, this book guides you through rejuvenation, basic food ideas, the prevention of disease, sprouts, stocking your kitchen, shopping and storage and weekly menu charts.

4 MENTAL AND SPIRITUAL FITNESS

Introduction

Down through the ages, thousands of books have been written about psychology and spirituality reflecting the fascination these fields hold for us. As I have discussed previously, total well being consists of body, mind and spirit. We have looked at the body component of total well being and we now need to address the mind and spirit as it relates to our emotional well being. I am most interested in interpretations of psychology and spirituality that make it possible for us to alter our patterns of behavior to create healthier lifestyles. In other words, those ways of looking at ourselves and the world around us that enable us to change. Since this book is all about change, it will help to examine those concepts or principles we can use as tools to facilitate that process.

NOTE:
"Change is the law of life. And those who look only to the past or the present are sure to miss the future."

John F. Kennedy, 1963

Psychology

During this process of moving toward total well being, I encourage patients to follow what M. Scott Peck, M.D. calls the **Road Less Traveled,**[1] that is, psychotherapy. Years ago, the gold standard for psychotherapy was through a heightened awareness of our unconscious, or psychoanalysis. Because this approach is long, arduous and expensive, it is not practical for

NOTE:
. . . our unconscious indisputably reigns over our motivations and, therefore, our actions.

the majority of us. Yet, dealing with our unconscious is necessary if we are to gain the integrity of personality necessary for positive change to take place. After all, our unconscious indisputably reigns over our motivations and, therefore, our actions.

If you are experiencing difficulty in changing some unwanted behaviors, another option is to take part in individual or group psychotherapy. It can be difficult to find a professional who is most suited to your unique problems and sensitivities, as well as someone with whom you feel comfortable communicating. The best way to find a good "match" is to get referrals from your physician, or by word of mouth from people you trust. Ask for an interview before committing yourself, your time and your money. Be wary of quick answers, avoid those who give guarantees and question someone who suggests that therapy needs to last for years. Your most important guide is to follow your intuition. "Does this person really care about my well being?"

Most people interested in behavioral change do not need a psychiatrist, that is a medical doctor who deals with chemical imbalances or diseases of the emotions and mind, and who usually prescribes drugs. Rather, I recommend a therapist who may be a psychologist, clinical social worker, counselor or minister. These people are trained to guide you through the process of wellness and to help with the healing of emotional pain.

Unfortunately, many people are reluctant to enter into professional therapy. Maybe it's the stigma associated with being seen by a "shrink." Heaven forbid that those societal judgments are still with us. More likely than not, however, people avoid therapy because they are unwilling to probe their inner fears in order to take a look at and change the way they deal with their past.

The Switch

One of the most puzzling questions I've ever encountered is, "How do you get people to change?" After years of trying, my response is, you DON'T, until that person is ready. This is frustrating, because it's usually obvious when people want to change their lives but don't seem to do it. Too often they need to "hit bottom" or have some "crisis" before they are willing to take action. It's a shame to see people struggle and suffer for so long.

NOTE:
"How do you get people to change?"

Fortunately, I am seeing more and more patients who get this wake up call while there is still time to salvage their health and, in some instances, totally reverse their condition and get on the road to recovery. The journey requires patience and commitment. After all, most people didn't get where they are without a long course of excessive physical abuse and neglect.

A Lady Who Enjoyed Theater

This wake up call to better health is exemplified by a lady I saw a few years ago. She was in her fifties and suffered from a severe weakness in her heart that left her unable to walk a block, constantly short of breath and chronically fatigued. She was on a multitude of medications, had serious heart rhythm disturbances, high blood cholesterol levels and diabetes. Worse, she compounded all those medical problems by weighing over three hundred pounds. Her life was miserable, with a grave prognosis . . . about a year to live.

She entered our weight loss and exercise program and within a year had lost over 100 pounds! She is down to one medicine and no longer has high cholesterol or diabetes. She is now walking on a treadmill for over 30 minutes. She looks and feels great!

NOTE:

*Finally, I decided
to take charge
of my own
life, to take
responsibility
for me.*

I asked her, "What was it that triggered you to turn your life around?" She started out with reminiscences like, "I love the theater and used to go only during matinees when I could reserve and hide in the big corner seats." She carried on "You have no idea what it means to me to be able to go to the theater now, in the evening, and sit anywhere I want." I gently persisted, "But, what caused you to switch inside?" She gave that some thought and finally said, "You know, all my life I went around blaming other people for what was happening to me. Finally, I decided to take <u>charge</u> of my own life, to take <u>responsibility</u> for me. Now, my life is totally different . . . I have a life!"

Triggers

This is a typical scenario, although the trigger, that "wake up call," may not need to be so dramatic. Take other patients of mine like the middle aged man who has a little memory loss due to atherosclerosis of the tiny blood vessels in his brain. Or, the overweight, out of shape executive who falls asleep during "boardroom conferences." These are the kinds of people who are beginning to take charge of their lives and make lifestyle changes toward total well being. They have come to our Institute for help because they have finally made the commitment to <u>change</u> their lives.

Still Stuck? Get Help!

If your triggers are not enough for you, but you are still stuck and want to change, get some "psychological" help to find out why you are not willing to take responsibility for your own life. Perhaps, you don't think you need it, deserve it or have the time, money and desire for formal therapy. Fortunately, there are many personal growth and development resources available to you. I will recommend a number of these and guide you through other processes that work for many of my patients.

Any of these resources may stimulate you to seek a more professional course or may provide you with the tools and techniques you need to take action. No matter what technique or level of help you choose, the important thing is to enable yourself to take action . . . to change self destructive behaviors to constructive behaviors that will allow you to, as the inspirational mythologist Joseph Campbell would say, "Follow your bliss."[2] That simply means caring enough about yourself to do what it takes to make healthy choices for yourself.

NOTE:
Care enough about yourself to do what it takes to make healthy choices for yourself.

Facing the unknown creates fear which can paralyze us. Yet, humans can make dramatic changes in their lives! For example, psychological experiments show that when people are subjected to something over and over again like criticism, unacceptable ideas or even physical abuse, they begin to accept it. This is known as the mirror exposure effect. Indeed, some people even begin to like the actions forced upon them despite the objectionable characteristics of such actions. We are amazingly adaptable creatures. The trick, however, is for us to use external forces in order to make changes from within. And the best way to change is to take deliberate and reasonable steps from where you are to where you want to be. You can do it!

Reasonable Transition

I tell my patients there are three steps you need to take in order to change; 1) Create a Vision, 2) Become Educated, and 3) Take Action! Of course, the last step is the most difficult, and frequently, we will enter into the first two just to fool our inner selves that we are doing something.

How many times have you heard someone say, "I'm going to lose weight one of these days," or, "You know, I'm going to write a book some day." That phrase "going to" is about as paralyzing as "if only." What a difference it makes in peoples lives when they <u>take</u> <u>action</u>! There are many different techniques that work to help people take action which I will discuss. Portions of this may seem far out to some of you, but I encourage you to read with an open mind because one of these approaches will work for you. Above all, know that the answers to your questions are within you.

This reminds me of a patient I interviewed recently. He was stuck on the fact that intellectually he knew what he needed to do in order to lose weight but just couldn't do it. "I've been through all the programs and know how to lose weight," he said. "I just don't understand why I stop at fast food restaurants, gorge myself, and then go home and eat another meal." I suggested that no weight management program would ever help him maintain his long term weight goals until he got to the underlying issues causing his behavior. After some seemingly non-productive discussion, we were walking down the hall together. He suddenly turned to me and said, "You know, maybe I'm just afraid of being successful." Wow! In just those few moments, he was beginning to find answers within himself and had progressed light years down his path.

Create a Vision

As you start down your path, consider where you want to end. This is crucial since your vision is a projection of your belief system. In all the resources that I have researched on personal growth and development, including lectures, tapes and books, there is always one key to success. Goals! You have to set goals. What do you really want?

Clearly, the majority of successful people set down their goals as a first step toward success. Just as clearly, the minority of people are not successful because they did not create a vision of what their goals are. Because this is such an important step, I urge everyone to pick up goal-setting books and tapes written by inspirational authors such as Napoleon Hill, Tony Robbins, Zig Ziglar and others. Look through the Nightingale Conant catalogue for these and other authors (1).

But don't wait. Begin now with these simple suggestions.

Set Goals

Crystallize your vision by first creating short term goals. Make them very specific, realistic and something that you can achieve within a few weeks. Next, develop your longer range goals, goals which could take you one to two years to achieve. Be specific about end points and accomplishment dates.

Imagine, in as much detail as you can, what you want to feel like and look like, both in the short-term and long-term. Your long range goals may seem unrealistic now, but they will become more and more achievable as you accomplish your short-term goals.

Post your short-term goals in places where they will provide you with constant reminders, such as on your bathroom mirror, or your refrigerator door, and place them in your wallet or purse. For example, "I will exercise for 20 minutes on Monday, Wednesday and Friday for three weeks" or "I will eat no desserts for one month." Change your goals as often as necessary to suit you. Let them work for you. Rewrite them to be just as specific as the original ones.

NOTE:
. . . the majority of successful people set down their goals as a first step toward success.

Take time now to fill out your short-term and long-term goals in Table 4.1 and 4.2, then transfer them to stickers and post them around your home environment. I know that this exercise may seem elementary, but it's these simple habits that get us redirected along a different path.

Table 4.1

GOALS : SHORT-TERM

Short-Term	
Goals	Accomplishment Date
_____	_____
_____	_____
_____	_____
_____	_____
_____	_____
_____	_____
_____	_____
_____	_____
_____	_____
_____	_____
_____	_____

Table 4.2
GOALS : LONG-TERM

Long-Term

Goals	Accomplishment Date
_____	_____
_____	_____
_____	_____
_____	_____
_____	_____
_____	_____
_____	_____
_____	_____
_____	_____
_____	_____
_____	_____

Become Educated

The next step is to become educated about those topics and techniques that will allow you to accomplish your goals. In a sense, you're in the process of education by obtaining and reading this book at this moment. To improve your physical fitness, start with the Practical Applications section in Chapter 2, then use the companion manual to this book, **Total Well Being Through Physical Fitness,** as your personal trainer. If you commit to the basic principles laid out in Chapter 3, "Nutrition," you will also begin to improve and master your eating habits. For those of you who wish to go beyond this chapter on psychological and spiritual growth, I have included many resources that can assist in changing your life.

Resources for Help

These resources cover a wide range of methods to attain mastery over the changes you wish to make. There are a number of personal growth and development organizations that provide literature and workshops to improving and enhancing your psychological and spiritual awareness. The basic philosophy of these groups has come a long way from the early days of personal growth seminars. Today's approach is far more nurturing and uses varied and credible techniques to stimulate your awareness. Many of them offer weekend retreats for people of all ages and socio-economic strata who want short, but intense exposure to ways of altering their behavior through greater awareness of their behavior patterns.

Keep in mind, however, that this type of organized emotional commitment, can create a transitory sense of euphoria or well being. Personal growth is an ongoing process. It's not like you attend one seminar and then you are "fixed." Therefore, it is important for you to find out if these organizations provide professional referrals and continued support. For example, many of them welcome volunteer assistance at subsequent meetings which can keep the momentum of your growth process on track.

On the other hand, your goal with any of these groups is to enhance your personal growth and development, not turn your personal power and energy over to someone else. For some people, the need to be a part of a greater entity . . . to be parented again . . . can result in cultism or total emotional commitment to another person. This transfer of needs and emotions to another, instead of empowering yourself from within, is completely counter to the self-help and growth I am describing here. Just as your nutritional well being depends on feeding your body with a diet of living foods, and not just the vitamin of the month, your psychological well being depends on feeding your psyche with true self awareness which comes from within, not from the guru of the month.

Turn to the resources at the end of this chapter for information on organizations (2-5) and institutes 6-8). I've discussed those which I have personally experienced and, therefore, can recommend. They will get you started on your journey ahead.

Taking Action

Once you have created your vision and have gained the knowledge you need to accomplish your goals, you are ready to take action. This is where most people get stuck, and there are a lot of ready-made distractions that help us stay stuck. The classic rationalization is that we need to take care of other people, our families or dutifully dedicate ourselves to our work. Let's admit it, change is scary. In reality, as selfish as it may sound, if we take care of ourselves first, and achieve total well being, we will be in a

NOTE:
Your goal is to enhance your personal growth and development, not turn your personal power and energy over to someone else.

much better position to enjoy our lives <u>and</u> serve others.

Once you have taken action, it's important to maintain a steady path. It seems that learning anything new is fraught with plateaus and setbacks. Many of us follow the process of change by taking two steps forward and one step backward. The pathway to success is often delayed or detoured by barriers and challenges to our most sincere intentions for change. Simply understanding this helps. That's what learning is all about, but all along you are moving in the right direction . . . toward total well being. Here is where three techniques can help a great deal; 1) Develop support systems, 2) Find role models and 3) Keep track of your progress with benchmarks.

Support Systems

A good example of how you can develop support systems was described by one of my more successful patients. She joined a health club where a friend of hers had been working out for some time. She signed up for nutrition classes at a local health food store, which provided her with inspiration and a way to meet supportive, health conscious friends. Another example of how social interaction with others can help you occurs daily in our Institute. The participants in our adult fitness program have an 80% attendance rate. This is because they exercise as a class, and the group dynamics serve as a support system.

You can enroll your family and friends into supporting your vision by sharing your goals with them. You will find some people who are very supportive even if they don't choose to live or eat like you do. Be aware, however, of those close to you who may try to sabotage your efforts.

Saboteurs

This phenomenon often happens to people embarked on a weight loss program. Characteristically, my weight loss patients have total support from their family and friends until they begin to reach their weight goals. Countless times, I have heard how, at first friends, and then family make comments such as, "You've lost enough weight, haven't you?" Or, "You don't need to lose any more weight, do you?" Then they proceed to, "Gosh, you look so thin and tired. Are you sure you're feeling OK?" You may ask yourself what is the purpose of their discouragement?

NOTE:
Your success at change only highlights the failures of those who sabotage you.

The simple explanation is that saboteurs are using a basic defense mechanism called projection. To them, your success at change only highlights their failures. They project their deficiencies on you in hopes that you will be vulnerable and stop whatever positive changes you are making that they are not able to accomplish themselves. Or, if you look and feel better, they fear that you may not continue to like them or need them. Be aware of these subtle dynamics going on around you, and don't let yourself be distracted from reaching your goal.

The best way to handle this type of behavior is to reflect upon it with care and compassion. Do not take what they say personally. Instead, trust that they are on their <u>right</u> path, and <u>you</u> stay resolute on your path.

Role Models

Role models can be a tremendous source of support and motivation. Surround yourself with books, audio tapes and videotapes, activities and creative visual art forms that support the plan you outlined in your goals. Pick out some inspirational tapes and listen to them in the morning or while driving (1). I find tapes to be both motivating and inspiring. If I am down or discouraged, they help encourage me, and I often feel refreshed and invigorated after listening to them.

Whom do you know socially that you admire and respect? Who in the business community do you look up to? Surround your self with these people. Ask them questions. Find out how they live and what motivates them.

NOTE:

"Our greatest glory is not in never falling, but in rising every time we fall."

Confucius, 550-478 B.C.

By using various modeling techniques like these, you learn that defeat can be used as an opportunity. Defeat is like the issue of good and bad, there has to be bad in order for good to exist. Likewise, defeat must exist, otherwise there would be no such thing as success! Over the years, I've heard athletes say time and again, that success does not come to those unwilling to fail. The willingness to fail, and learn from it, is a part of achieving success. Accept defeat without all the personal judgments we usually associate with it, then use it as a springboard to move on to greater accomplishments.

Benchmark

Keeping track of your progress is just as valuable as setting goals. Reflecting upon the overall progress that you've made and the new resources you've discovered, can give you the confidence you need to maintain your new behaviors and to make new commitments to change. The best way to accurately reflect on your progress is to benchmark the changes you've made as you proceed along your path.

Keep track of your progress. Create tables and charts that reflect your progress in behavioral changes such as diet, physical fitness or stress reduction. Ask your doctor and other health care providers to help you undergo periodic tests such as blood tests, exercise tests and fitness evaluations. Then, use this information to look at and judge the changes you have made. Above all, do not be discouraged by the plateaus and set backs. They are only temporary. Keep the bigger picture in mind. Soon, you'll be feeling, great!

"Addictions"

We all have our "addictions," that is, an uncontrollable craving for something that ultimately works against us. Like any psychological concept, there are degrees of addiction from enthusiastic devotion, to obsessive compulsion, to complete loss of control. The consequences to our health are equally graded from mild to critical. The most common system we use to defend our addictions is rationalization. We use reasonable and logical arguments to explain our attitudes and behaviors to ourselves and to others. Indeed, such defense mechanisms are commonly used so we can remain comfortable with life . . . to keep going on an even keel. However, when we maintain an addictive behavior over an extended period of time, the effect can be devastating to our health. We eventually get stuck in a rut that can become a vicious cycle, preventing us from developing into and becoming the person we were truly meant to be.

NOTE:
One of the first steps to getting out of this rut is to . . . understand that we choose our addictions.

One of the first steps to getting out of this rut is to own up to our addictions and . . . this may sound a bit harsh . . . understand that we <u>choose</u> our addictions. Who, for example, sat you in a chair, tied your hands behind your back and force fed you greasy, sugary foods? Who chained you to a life of inactivity on the couch in front of televised programming aimed at the level of a third grader? Who dragged you back to the office for another day of drudgery?

In order to change, we must start with the realization that it is our own behaviors and actions that lead us to this addictive behavior. We can blame ourselves. You must realize that you are ultimately responsible for this situation, and you are the only one that can effect change. There are many people and organizations to help you, but only <u>you</u> can take the first step toward change.

This raises a key concept that can help jolt you out of this stagnant cycle. Simply ask yourself how it benefits you to choose your addiction again, and again and again.

A Powerful Process

This question forms the basis of one of the simplest yet most powerful, processes I've encountered in helping people initiate change in their lives. If you are ready, honest with yourself and willing to do some deep soul searching, carefully read and answer the following question:

"How does it serve me to choose to_____?"

Fill in the blank with whatever issue you think might be keeping you from achieving your full potential as a human being. For example, many of my patients want to lose weight, so they would fill in the blank with "overeat." You might choose to "eat poorly," "let my body deteriorate by not exercising," "be a workaholic," "smoke cigarettes," "drink too much," etc.

What's Your First Reaction?

The first reaction most people have to this question is puzzled indignation, "Well, it doesn't <u>serve</u> me in any way to be overweight!" And I certainly do not <u>choose</u> it!"

That's a natural reaction, but it doesn't take much logic to convince someone that they have not been forced into their actions. With a little discussion, most people begin to understand that, indeed, they do choose their own behavior.

Then, I ask them if it seems reasonable that, as a rational, mature, intelligent human being, they would choose to do anything if it did not benefit them in <u>some</u> <u>way</u> or another. It helps, at this point to rephrase the question by asking, "What does it do for you to choose to," or "What do you get out of choosing to _____?"

NOTE:
Would you choose to do anything if it did not benefit you in <u>some</u> <u>way</u> or another?

One of My Weight Loss Patients

By then, most people begin to get the gist of the process. As an example, a typical conversation with one of my weight loss patients who wants to stop overeating may go something like this:

Q: "How do you think it could serve you to overeat?"
A: "Well, it helps me deal with stress, and I feel better."

Q: "And then, what do you get out of choosing to over eat?"
   Pause
A: "Ah, well, I get sick."

Q: "Good recognition. And, how does it serve you to choose to get sick?"

Pause

A: "I don't know."

Q: "Well, if you did know. . . how could it possibly serve you to become sick?"

A: "When I get sick, I get depressed."

Q: "Good, you're doing fine. And, how does it benefit you to choose to get depressed?"

A: "When I get depressed, I feel isolated and withdrawn."

Q: "How does it serve you to choose to become withdrawn?"

A: "I don't have to face anyone else, and I can hide."

Once someone catches on to this line of questioning, "How does it serve you to choose to," or "How do you feel as a result of what you choose to do?" . . . the answers begin to flow more easily, and along with it comes an incredible amount of self awareness. It doesn't take long to get into the feeling responses, and that usually means we are getting close to the heart of the matter.

Let's review what has just happened by using a diagram.

I break this scenario out into two spirals, Figure 4.1. Initially, there is the immediate pleasure principle where people eat as a way of handling anxiety. This is not surprising, since "oral gratification," in the general sense of the word, is a strong instinct we developed and had reinforced during our infancy. I've reluctantly learned over the years that those people who are not yet ready or willing to commit to change are better left alone in this dead end loop. But, if you want to encourage awareness on their part, keep asking the same question. No addicting behavior leads to gratification without its consequences. The consequences then take us into the second spiral.

The second spiral gets us into a downward cycle where one behavior or feeling reinforces the next. In the example above, it was sickness that triggered depression, which led to isolation, withdrawal and finally "protection."

Figure 4.1
THE SPIRAL OF SELF AWARENESS

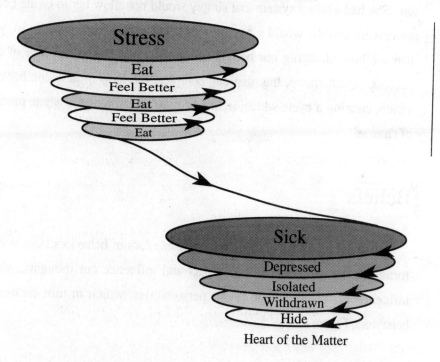

Heart of the Matter

This reflective process peels away the layers of rationalization and subterfuge like the leaves of an artichoke, to get down to the "heart of the matter." And, in my experience, the heart of the matter is the same for every one of us. Before I develop that thought to it's conclusion, however, I urge you to spend some time with this process dealing with your "addictions."

You have the answers inside of you to peel away the layers right down to your bottom line. Take advantage of looking inside yourself and finding out how you benefit from choosing to . . . .

Our Belief Systems

NOTE:

"He does not believe that does not live according to his belief."

Thomas Fuller, M.D., 1732

Our bottom line is based upon our belief systems. For example, one of my patients believed she was not capable of being successful at weight loss. She had failed so many times that, on a very deep level, she had given up. She had a belief system that simply would not allow her to create being successful, and she would sabotage herself and create more failure. So, you can see how changing our beliefs about ourselves lies at the core of our success. Furthermore, this step can complete the loop from action back to vision, creating a cycle which, in and of itself, reinforces the whole process of change.

Beliefs

Our beliefs are ultimately responsible for our behaviors. Our beliefs formulate our attitudes, which impact and influence our thoughts, which influence the development of our personalities, which in turn create our behaviors, Figure 4.2.

Figure 4.2
THE CREATION OF OUR BELIEF SYSTEMS

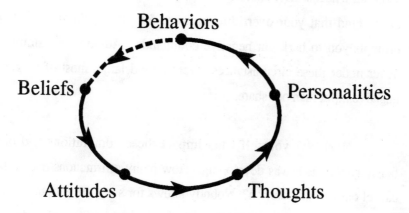

Since your belief system is at the root or your behavior, it's time to make some changes!

How did we develop our belief systems in the first place? In general, it is formed from the knowledge and experiences we have up to age six. As newborns, we receive information through our senses. The earliest information is conveyed through touch, taste and smell. As our brains develop, the information comes more in the from of visual and verbal cues. Later on, as our cognitive abilities develop, information comes primarily through verbal communication.

Affirmations and Admonitions

What information went into conditioning our belief systems? Regardless of the sensory modality, two kinds of information shape our beliefs; affirmations and admonitions. Affirmations are messages that carry positive assertions. Admonitions carry messages that express authoritative advice or warnings. As you were growing up, how many admonitions did you receive for every affirmation? Most people say 80 to 20 or 90 to 10. This isn't necessarily unnatural. For example, if you are a parent, you understand that your overriding concern for your children's safety often prompts you to bark out negative commands. Admonitions simply work better under these circumstances. Yet, by and large, most of us got more negative input than our share.

Next, ask yourself what impact these admonitions had on your belief system as it was developing. How many affirmations does it take to cancel out one admonition? Nobody knows for sure, but people often say it takes 10, 50 or even a 100 affirmations to negate one single admonition. Regardless of the numbers, research clearly demonstrates that our belief systems are primarily created from negative stimuli!

At the Heart of the Matter

NOTE:
... the heart of the matter is the same for every one of us ... low self esteem!

This is very powerful information and it brings me back to the process I described above and the heart of the matter. It explains why our core issues, why as we peel away the layers around us, the heart of the matter is the same for every one of us . . . low self esteem! When people are honest and willing to search deeply enough, the answer they almost always find is, "I don't really love myself." Many of our attitudes, thoughts, personalities, and behaviors reinforce our deep down beliefs that we are not worth behaving any differently! Our actions protect and reinforce these beliefs. We have low self esteem and do not love ourselves enough to take care of ourselves and show the world how magnificent we really are.

This takes me back to the classic concept of Eric Fromm when he wrote in the **Art of Loving** that we must learn to love ourselves before we can love anyone else.[3] I believe that adopting this concept can promote the change we are looking for. We can take action if we learn to restructure our beliefs about who we are and appreciate the unique God given gifts we possess.

Poor self esteem lies at the root of our belief systems that, through an elaborate series of defense mechanisms, winds its way up to destructive behavior. Can your behavior be changed? Yes, if you change your belief system. Can your belief system be changed? Yes, after all, it was formed in the first place!

You Can Change!

When I first considered changing my basic beliefs, I thought, "Don't fool with Mother Nature!" Then, it occurred to me that my nature had already been fooled with. And, if we want to change our belief systems, let's do it the same way that they were created in the first place. The difference being that this time we can load the stimuli with affirmations instead of admonitions!

NOTE:
. . . we can load the stimuli with affirmations instead of admonitions!

Repeat Affirmations

Affirmations are positive visualizations of who you are and who you want to be. Make lists of these affirmations and post them in places where you will be constantly reminded of those qualities in yourself. Every night in a notebook you keep by your bedside, write down, "Seven things I love about myself." At first this may be difficult, but it gets easier and more believable the longer you do it. Review your notebook every three months and you will find repetitious affirmations that represent who <u>you</u> really are.

This alone could change your life!

There are a number of commercial self talk and motivational tapes available (9). For many people, listening to one of them for positive verbal affirmations helps their self confidence and motivation to stay on track with the changes they want to make in their lives. It certainly works for me.

Every morning I have a tape recorder blaring away in the bathroom carrying on about what a great guy I am. Although embarrassing at first, this constant positive reinforcement has helped me realize I'm all right after all. As I continue to grow, I occasionally find myself disagreeing with the content of the taped message and rewrite the information to better suit me. Then I record myself saying the new affirmations and listen to these personalized motivational tapes.

There are also subliminal tapes. They contain repetitive affirmations recorded at such speeds and frequencies that you hear only the overriding sounds of soothing music or sounds of nature. Their effectiveness is based on the premise that the messages reach your unconscious brain without being filtered through the <u>conscious</u> brain. Use only those tapes that provide you in writing with the messages or affirmations to see if you agree with what they say before you play the tapes. I particularly recommend Sound R_X which teams up Stephen Halpern, a musician, with John Bradshaw, a psychologist experienced in self-help psychology (10).

Avoid Negatives

Another way to change your belief system is to avoid negatives. Every time you catch yourself saying a negative, say "cancel" out loud. Encourage your close friends, family and receptive colleagues to point out any negative self talk. Ask them to give you a friendly "cancel" when they catch you at it.

Use "I"

An additional suggestion I make to patients is to shift their thinking and self talk into the first person. Speak for yourself. Use "I" instead of "you" when you talk. In the beginning this may seem awkward. Most of us feel uncomfortable using "I" when speaking about emotions and feelings. It's much easier to hide behind the generic "you" than to face our own feelings. When I began using the first person, I often felt emotions I had never experienced before. However, as I became more accustomed to listening and learning about myself, I also became more accepting and appreciative of who I really am. Next time you find yourself arguing with a colleague or family member, try saying, "I don't like to talk to you this way." Sense what awareness that language brings up for you.

NOTE:
It's much easier to hide behind the generic "you" than to face our own feelings.

Change your beliefs with what ever approaches work for you. Your attitudes, thoughts, personality and finally, at last, your behaviors will change. Remember, total well being is an integrated balance of our physical psychological and spiritual well being. As you improve in any realm the others also improve. This is particularly true between our mental and spiritual natures.

Spirituality

Writing about spirituality is a daunting task because there are so many different approaches to exploring and achieving spiritual well being. Moreover, people have often made up their minds as to what they will and will not believe. Their beliefs range from orthodox religions to the sectarian and new age philosophies. Yet, Spirit is as essential a component of total well being as Body and Mind.

Therefore, I'll discuss this topic from an approach based upon my personal, academic and professional experiences. After all, experiences are the only point of view anyone can offer. It is not my intention to convince you to adopt my views, I simply want to awaken your thinking about spiritual matters, or have you solidify your present beliefs.

The Higher Power

I am constantly reminded of the miracle of life, every time I study the intricate, interrelated details of human biochemistry, physiology and anatomy. What a mind-boggling experience; and our knowledge is still only primitive! Fishing in my small boat miles off the coast of Miami, bobbing up and down in the swells of the Gulf stream, I become absorbed in a huge panorama of blue hues from the ocean and sky. This evokes a sense of spirituality in me that goes way beyond my intellectual comprehension. These experiences unequivocally convince me that there is a creative force responsible for existence. Call it what you will, The Creator, The Universal Being, Oneness, God, or, as I do, The Higher Power, something's out there, somewhere.

It stands to reason that humans gain spirituality by connecting with that power. And, how do we connect? It must be through that unique feature which distinguishes human beings from other animals . . . the cerebral cortex. This highly developed portion of our brains has the capability of memory, cognition, creativity and imagination. Together, I call these collective capabilities the "mind" or "consciousness." As we develop a higher, more enlightened consciousness, we are better able to connect with the higher universal power and, therefore, develop greater spirituality.

Our Minds

In order for our minds to function completely, however, both the right and left cerebral hemispheres must communicate with each other. We are able to develop a higher consciousness when there is neural integration between the left and the right cerebral hemispheres. There is just one problem: the two sides of the brain are physically separated by an anatomical barrier, a fibrous tissue called the corpus collosum, Figure 4.3.

NOTE:
. . . both the right and left cerebral hemispheres must communicate with each other.

Figure. 4.3
DIVISION OF THE TWO HEMISPHERES
By the Corpus Collosum

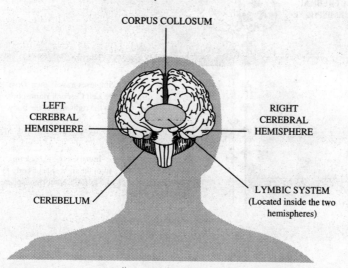

CORPUS COLLOSUM

LEFT CEREBRAL HEMISPHERE

RIGHT CEREBRAL HEMISPHERE

CEREBELUM

LYMBIC SYSTEM
(Located inside the two hemispheres)

The corpus collosum blocks nerve impulses from communicating between the left and right side of our brains, thereby interfering with the integration we need in order to develop our minds, our higher consciousness and, thus, our spirituality. However, communication can be established between both sides of the brain. This occurs as nerve impulses move <u>down</u> through our bodies and <u>back up</u> to our brains. This crucial mechanism re-emphasizes the importance for us to "listen to our bodies."

Integration of Both Hemispheres

Impulses move from one hemisphere down through the base of the brain where they cross over to the other side of the body, and then on to the bodily functions, Figure 4.4. From there, sensory impulses return by crossing back over in the spinal cord and returning back up to the same cerebral hemisphere.

Figure 4.4
IMPULSES CROSS OVER
From One Side of the Brain to the Other

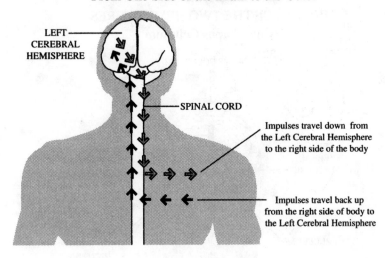

LEFT CEREBRAL HEMISPHERE

SPINAL CORD

Impulses travel down from the Left Cerebral Hemisphere to the right side of the body

Impulses travel back up from the right side of body to the Left Cerebral Hemisphere

Perhaps you are aware of the fact that the left side of the brain controls the right side of the body and vice versa. For example, when someone has a stroke on the left side of his or her brain, the right side of his or her body may become paralyzed. So, how do we get the integration between the two hemispheres?

This has to do with two other portions of the brain, the cerebellum and the limbic system. The cerebellum is located in the lower brain and controls our bodies' balance and coordination. The limbic system is deep in the middle of the brain where emotions are generated and integrated.

As sensory impulses return back up to the brain from the body, they travel through cerebellum, Figure 4.5. The cerebellum sends nerve impulses back up to both hemispheres in order to coordinate both sides of the body as we move. Stop and think about how intricately balanced both sides of your body are as you walk, get up out of a chair, comb your hair, etc.

NOTE:
The cerebellum connects both sides of the brain by sending nerve impulses back up to both hemispheres.

Figure 4.5
THE CONNECTION BETWEEN THE HEMISPHERES
Through the Cerebellum

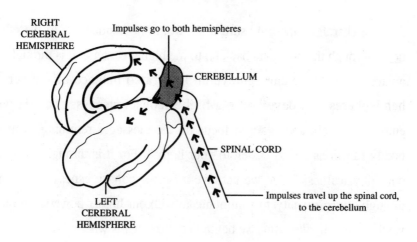

RIGHT CEREBRAL HEMISPHERE

Impulses go to both hemispheres

CEREBELLUM

SPINAL CORD

Impulses travel up the spinal cord, to the cerebellum

LEFT CEREBRAL HEMISPHERE

NOTE:

The limbic system connects both sides of the brain by secreting neurohormones that circulate to both hemispheres.

Impulses also travel back up from the body and pass through the limbic system, Figure 4.6. One way that emotions are integrated between both sides of the brain is that the limbic system secretes neurohormones into the blood stream which circulate to both hemispheres. Once again we see how messages from the body find their way back to the opposite hemisphere which bridges the gap between the left and right cerebral hemispheres.

Figure 4.6
THE CONNECTION BETWEEN THE HEMISPHERES
Through the Limbic System

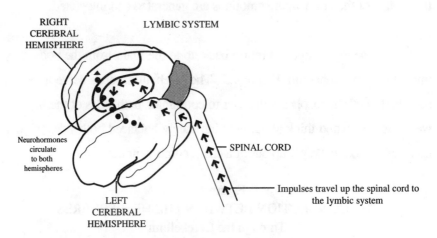

Therefore, the only sure route from one hemisphere to the other is <u>down</u> through the body and <u>back up</u> to the higher centers. It is through body awareness that we can achieve an integrated balance of the cerebral hemispheres . . . developing a higher consciousness. This is why I emphasize again and again to focus on the messages returning from your bodily functions . . . to "listen to your body." For it is through listening to our "physicalness," that we achieve a higher consciousness allowing us, through our spirituality, to communicate with our higher powers. In fact, as we listen <u>within</u> ourselves, we begin to realize that is where the power is.

The Power Within Us

The power within us is our salvation to freedom. That is, as we turn our lives over to the control of the power within us, we become free from the burden of self control. That doesn't mean we have no responsibility. Rather, our responsibility is simply to follow the power within us. In this way, the creative power of the universe lives through each of us, and we can become one with the creator.

NOTE:
"You're not free until you've been made captive by supreme belief."
Marianne Moore, 1951

As you internalize your understanding of the power within you, your intuition gives you the ability to make judgments about your life. As your understanding becomes clearer and more meaningful to you, your communication with the power of your understanding becomes more direct and more confident. This is what personal power is all about. Once you tap into your own personal power, all of those external powers, instead of becoming dictates, become resources to you. The power within you is your source to know and fulfill the goals for which you have been created.

To many of you, discussions like this may sound far out, inappropriate or uncomfortable. However, the rewards of this type of reflection are infinite and particularly pertinent to our rational western world. Be persistent and patient because, although it may take time, the benefits of understanding the power within you could make the difference in your achieving total well being.

Summary

I suggest psychotherapy down the road less traveled. At the very least, use the other resources I've discussed to assist you. Look for the switch inside that will permit you to commit to change. Set your goals, learn what you need to do and take action! Don't be afraid to look inside yourself. <u>You</u> have the answers. Listen for them. Use what works for you and change your beliefs . . . your behaviors will surely change.

Integrate your mind by listening to your body. As you enhance your mind and develop a higher consciousness, tap into and turn your trust over to the power within you. That <u>power</u> is your source of freedom. The freedom to communicate who you truly are.

Practical Applications

Deep Breathing

The single, most powerful relaxation technique you can perform is to consciously focus on deep breathing. It's easy to learn, quick and simple to do, and provides immediate benefits. Breathing is controlled by our autonomic nervous systems which regulate all of our stress response mechanisms. Think of the ways our breathing is related to our emotions, the startled gasp; the shallow, rapid breathing of fear; the trembling breath of anger; the halted, sobbing breathing of grief; the slow, labored breath of depression; and the sigh of relief. Yet, we can consciously control our breathing. In so doing, we modulate the way our autonomic nervous systems impact on our bodies, and we achieve an overall calming effect. This goes along with the idea I presented earlier about listening to your "physicalness" as you go down into your body and back up to integrate both cerebral hemispheres and enhance your consciousness.

> **NOTE:**
> *Deep breathing is easy to learn, quick and simple to do, and provides immediate benefits.*

Deep Breathing Exercise

- Sit upright in a chair.
- Breathe in through your nose for four counts.
- Inhale slowly and continuously.
- Fill your lower lungs by drawing your diaphragm down and pushing your abdomen out.
- Then, fill the middle part of your lungs by drawing your lower rib cage out and up.
- Finally, fill your upper lungs by raising your chest up and drawing your abdomen in.

- Hold your breath for six counts.
- Exhale through your mouth for eight counts.
- Completely empty your lungs by slightly squeezing in your abdomen and raising up your chest.
- This is one breath cycle. Repeat at least four times.

Notice that exhalation takes twice as long as inhalation, although the actual time you take for each cycle is irrelevant. However, the ratio of 4:6:8 is important. Some yoga masters also encourage holding the tip of your tongue against your inner gum behind your upper front teeth throughout the entire exercise. You may also find it easier to concentrate on your breathing by quietly inhaling and making a soft whooshing sound as you exhale.

After a little practice, this breathing exercise becomes automatic, and you will be amazed at how quickly and easily you will achieve a sense of well being.

Progressive Muscle Relaxation

Progressive muscle relaxation is the oldest, and most commonly practiced, clinical method of stress management and relaxation. This technique can be practiced lying down or sitting up in a chair. Begin by taking in a series of slow, deep breaths. Next, tense a specific group of muscles as tight as you can for about five seconds. Then, completely relax them for 15 to 20 seconds. Throughout the exercise, tune in to your body. Stay in touch with your breathing and sense that you breathe in positive energy and exhale tension. Begin with your feet and work up through your body to your head.

Progressive Muscle Relaxation Exercise

You can develop your own progression to suit the needs of your time and place. The following is a technique when lying down:

- Bend your toes up and flex your shins as tightly as you can. Release and breathe evenly.

- Curl your toes downward and tighten your calves. Relax, and sense any tingling in your legs and feet.

- Flex your thighs by pressing your heels down as far as you can. Notice the tension. Relax.

- Squeeze your thighs and buttocks as tightly as possible. Relax and feel the soothing heaviness in your legs.

- Tighten your stomach as hard as possible and press your back against the floor. Relax and imagine you can feel the organs inside your abdomen.

- Take in a deep breath. Keeping your abdomen relaxed, hold your breath and squeeze your chest tightly. Let the air flow out completely, then push out the last traces of air. Totally relax your body and let your breath come deeply, smoothly and comfortably.

- As you relax more deeply, sense that energizing air comes in and tension drains away with each exhalation.

- Squeeze your hands and forearms as tightly as you can. Release and feel any tingling sensation in your hands.

- Contract your biceps and triceps as much as possible. Relax, and feel the warmth in your arms.

- Shrug your shoulders up and scrunch your neck down, tighter and tighter. Release and feel the relaxation spread throughout your shoulders, neck and throat. Be aware that your body may feel like it's floating.

- Keeping your eyes and mouth closed, raise your forehead up and lower your jaw as far as you can. Contract the muscles in front of your neck. Relax and feel the tension inside your head melt away.

- Squint your eyes and squeeze every muscle in your face as tightly as you can. Relax, and feel a warm flush flow from the front to the back of your head. Perhaps chills trickle down your body.

- Breathe evenly and smoothly as you relax more and more deeply.

Meditation

NOTE:

Meditation is an extremely valuable tool to calm yourself, relax your muscles and quiet your mind.

The more I devote to the integration of the brain and the development of a higher conscious, the greater my understanding of the power within me and, therefore, my spirituality becomes. This requires listening to myself, which I call silent time. Many people call this meditation. For some people this time is spent in prayer, yet prayer creates a focus for the mind which is not the same as truly listening to the power within yourself. In today's fast-paced society, silent time is hard to come by for most people. It is, however, an extremely valuable tool to calm yourself, relax your muscles and quiet your mind. This peaceful state makes it easier for you to deal with the enormous stresses of everyday life.

The Time and Place

First of all, you need to make time and set it aside each day for this purpose. You may find that several short periods of time each day are more effective than one long period of time. Next, find a location where you can have complete privacy. Select a comfortable chair or pillows to sit on. Soft music, a vase of flowers, geometric shapes, or candles may enhance your ability to focus your mind . . . focus on "nothing." For many people, their quiet time is early morning before they get distracted by the day's events. I find that waking up and meditating during sunrise gives me a sense of peace within the hustle and bustle of this very busy world.

Mental Chatter

Once you've designated a time, don't be surprised at what you experience when you begin sitting in silence. Although your goal is total silence . . . the peace and serenity that come from communicating with your inner high power . . . it may take some time before you get there. What used to happen during the first moments of my silent time was always the same. I was bombarded with non-stop mental chatter in all forms and from all directions. The harder I tried to fight the mental chatter, the more dominant it became. However, if you just let the chatter happen, let your thoughts come and go, they will gradually become less and less dominating. In other words, by not judging, not analyzing, but simply by accepting your thoughts, they will soon cease their clamor for your attention. Ironically, the nothingness that you begin to listen to becomes the everything that you hear.

Another successful technique to enhance your concentration during silent time, is to mentally repeat a mantra or a series of syllables. Or, focus on your breathing as I described above. What happens to your emotions when you hold your breath? Obviously, you pen up your feelings and thoughts. Many say that release through the breath is the key to enlightenment. Some people find their first attempts at listening within are made easier with audio tapes that combine explanations with guided imagery (11).

Whatever techniques you adopt, this is your opportunity to tap into your mind, enhance your higher consciousness and communicate with your higher power. This is spirituality.

NOTE:
Ironically, the nothingness that you begin to listen to becomes the everything that you hear.

Resources

Nightingale Conant offers a wide variety of audio tapes, videotapes and books designed to enrich and change your life (1). They include works from experienced and trusted leaders in the fields of self-help and motivation for success.

There are a number of organizations around the country that offer weekend personal growth and development courses. These courses are gaining in popularity as a growing number of people are becoming more open to self-awareness and to realizing their full potential. Individuals who have chosen to participate in these courses or workshops report significant improvements in such areas as self-confidence, self esteem, interpersonal relationships, lowered job stress, a heightened sense of control in life, and a more positive and pleasurable range of events and experiences in their lives.

NOTE:
The processes utilized in these self help courses are amazing. Each exercise seems to get better and better in creating self awareness. . .

Many of these organizations have more advanced courses which may be longer and often require residence at their headquarters. The processes utilized in these courses are amazing. Each exercise seems to get better and better in creating self awareness, either directly through your own experience or vicariously from others. The workshops are taught by instructors trained and certified by the parent organization.

The introductory course of Avatar is taught in groups and is designed to help you explore your own consciousness and modify whatever you want to change (2). Avatar materials and workbooks are utilized to help the student achieve these goals. The Insight Transformation Seminars (3) and Lifespring courses (4) are usually conducted in large groups. The processes they use become more amazing as the experience progresses. UYO (Understanding Yourself and Others) is the introductory course provided by Global Relationship Centers and is perhaps the most intense experience, since the enrollment is limited, offering a greater opportunity for student participation (5).

There are a number of resident institutes that provide lectures, courses, seminars and workshops in all areas of well being. These facilities are often visited by the foremost lecturers and authors in their respective fields, as well as having an enlightened and experienced resident staff. The Esalen Institute in Big Sur California, in operation over thirty years, is open mid-September to mid-June (6). Their programs focus on areas of environmental design, transformative practice and theoretical work related to human potential. The Omega Institute for Holistic Studies is open during the summer months (7). Their curriculum is grouped into five overlapping areas, Self, Others, Expression, World and Spirit. The Kripalu Center for Yoga and Health is open year-round (8). They offer instruction in meditation, yogic breathing and Kripalu yoga. This is a type of yoga designed to allow you to encounter and release the physical, mental and emotional blocks that hold you back; a way to discover your true inborn potential.

Shad Helmstetter has developed a series of self-talk audio tapes that give you enthusiastic affirmations and non-stop encouragement to improve your self image and create internal motivation to accomplish specific goals (9). These are excellent tapes to have playing in the background as you carry on routine daily activities.

Of all the subliminal tapes available, I recommend the series from Steven Halpern and Sound R_X (10). Steve's music automatically evokes your body's relaxation response. This helps focus your subconscious mind on the carefully scripted affirmations, many of which are created in cooperation with John Bradshaw, Ph.D., lecturer, author and host of the PBS-TV series, *Homecoming*. The script is written out for each tape so you can inspect the exact affirmations which are being played.

Guided visual imagery is often helpful to the beginner in meditation. It offers a structure that helps focus your mind and minimize the distractions from mental chatter. The Monroe Institute uses certain sound combinations and frequencies to "induce distinct states of consciousness not ordinarily available to the human mind" (11). The Institute has week-long group seminars and an in-home exercise series on audio tape cassettes.

Epilogue

I hope you enjoyed reading this book nearly as much as I enjoyed preparing it for you. Indeed, I am grateful for what I've learned up to this point in my life. I turned my life around, feel the best that I've ever felt, and am excited to share this journey with you. I look around and see an unwell population, unhappiness in the faces of a lot of people of all ages. I yearn for them to make the switch inside that gives them the courage and commitment to be ready and willing to begin their journey to total well being.

> **NOTE:**
> *"Total Well Being is an integrated balance of Body, Mind and Spirit."*
>
> Jack E. Young, M.D, Ph.D.,
> 1994

The path that we need to take is simple. We all know deep down inside . . . intuitively . . . exactly what we must do to lead happy and full lives. We need to treat our physical bodies with the respect it deserves. We need to get rid of the sludge and poisons that irritate and raise havoc with the cells, tissues, organs, and the systems that make up our physical natures. We need to feed our bodies with optimal nutrition in order to function smoothly, to grow strong, to mature wisely and to age with grace. We need to exercise so that our tissues can develop strength and flexibility. We need to breathe in and deliver oxygen, the essence of life, to all of our cells so they can explode with bioenergy and our bodies can beam and radiate with exuberance. We need to integrate and balance all aspects of our brains; our intelligence, emotions and autonomic nervous functions and allow them to interact with our physical functions. We need to nurture our minds, develop a higher consciousness and communicate with the power within us!

I did say that this is simple. I admit it may not be easy. The external influences in our lives smother us in ways that counter all that we know is good for us. However, as we take these simple steps one at a time and improve our physical being, enhance our minds and communicate with our spirit, we will come to know the power within us. Then, if we are willing to trust that power, we can take in external energies and redirect them through that power back out to the world to create love and harmony everywhere. Welcome to the journey!

Bibliography
Resources and References

Chapter 1

Resources

(1). Hepner, J. O. and D. M. Hepner. **The Health Strategy Game. A Challenge for Reorganization and Management.** The C.V. Mosby Co., St. Louis, MO. 1973. ISBN: 0-8016-2144-5.

(2). Illich, I. **Medical Nemesis. The Expropriation of Health.** Pantheon Books, New York, NY. 1976. ISBN: 0-394-40225-1.

(3). Annis, E. R. **Code Blue. Health Care in Crisis.** Regnery Gateway, Washington, DC. 1993. ISBN: 0-89526-515-X.

(4). *An Agenda for Solving America's Health Care Crisis.* Task Force Report, NCPA Policy Report No. 151. Revised June 1991. ISBN: 0943802-54-7. National Center for Policy Analysis. 1265 N. Central Expressway, Suite 720, Dallas, TX, 75243. (214) 386 6272.

(5). American Holistic Medical Association. 4101 Lake Boone Trail, Suite 201, Raleigh, NC, 27607. (919) 787 5146. Fax (919) 787 4916.

(6). American College for Advancement in Medicine. 3121 Verdugo Dr., Suite 204, Laguna Hills, CA, 92653. (714) 583 7666. Fax (714) 455 9679.

(7). Physicians Committee for Responsible Medicine. 5100 Wisconsin Ave. NW, Suite 404, Washington, DC, 20017. (202) 686 2210. Fax (202) 686 2216.

References

(1). Bal, D. and S. Foerster. *Diet Strategies for Cancer Prevention.* Cancer. 1993; 72:1005-1010.

(2). Department of Health and Human Services. *The Health Consequences of Smoking.* Cancer: A Report of the Surgeon General. Rockville, MD. 1982.

(3). Sandler, R. S., et al. *Diet and Risk of Colorectal Adenomas: Macronutrients, Cholesterol, and Fiber.* J Natl Cancer Inst. 1993; 85:884-890.

(4). Barrett-Connor, E. *Dietary Fat, Calories and the Risk of Breast Cancer in Post Menopausal Women: A Prospective Population-Based Study.* J Am Coll Nutr. 1993; 12:390-399.

(5). Boyd, N. *Nutrition and Breast Cancer.* J Natl Cancer Inst. 1993; 85:6-7.

(6). Schachter, S. *Recidivism and Self-Cure of Smoking and Obesity.* Am Psychol. 1982; 37:436-444.

(7). Paffenbarger, R. S., et al. *Physical Activity, All-Cause Mortality, and Longevity of College Alumni.* N Engl J Med. 1986; 314:605-613.

(8). Hubert, H. B., et al. *Obesity as an Independent Risk Factor for Cardiovascular Disease: A 26-Year Follow-up of Participants in the Framingham Heart Study.* Circulation. 1983; 67:968-977.

Chapter 2

Resources

(1). Young, J. E. **Total Well Being Through Physical Fitness**. Tri Health, Inc. 1717 N Bayshore Dr., Suite 3936, Miami, FL, 33132. (1-800) DR YOUNG (379 6864).

References

(1). Paffenbarger, R. S., et al. *Physical Activity, All-Cause Mortality, and Longevity of College Alumni.* N Engl J Med. 1986; 314:605-613.

2. Baun, W. B., et al. *A Preliminary Investigation: Effect of a Corporate Fitness Program on Absenteeism and Health Care Cost.* J Occup Med. 1986; 28:18-22.

(3). Blair, S., et al. *A Public Health Intervention Model for Work-Site Health Promotion.* JAMA. 1986; 255:921-926.

(4). Spilman, M. A., et al. *Effects of a Corporate Health Promotion Program.* J Occup Med. 1986; 28:285-290.

(5). Van Camp, S. *Exercise-Related Sudden Death: Risks and Causes (Part 1 of 2).* Phys Sportsmed. 1988; 16:97-112.

(6.) Ibid.

(7). Mittleman, M. A., et al. *Triggering of Acute Myocardial Infarction by Heavy Physical Exertion: Protection Against Triggering by Regular Exertion.* N Engl J Med. 1993; 329:1677-1683.

(8). Willich, S. N., et al. *Physical Exertion as a Trigger of Acute Myocardial Infarction.* N Engl J Med. 1993; 329:1684-1690.

(9). Pouliot, M. C., et al. *Visceral Obesity in Men: Associations with Glucose Tolerance, Plasma Insulin and Lipoprotein Levels.* Diabetes. 1992; 41:826-834.

(10). Shimokata, H., et al. *Studies in the Distribution of Body Fat: I. Effects of Age, Sex and Obesity.* J. Gerontol. 1989; 44:M66-73.

Chapter 3

Resources

(1). Sorenson, M. **Mega Health**. Available from:
The National Institute of Fitness. 202 North Snow Canyon Road, Box 938,
Ivins, UT, 84738. (801) 673 4905.

(2). Pritikin, N. **The Pritikin Promise: 28 Days to a Longer,
Healthier Life.** Simon & Schuster, Inc. 1230 Avenue of the Americas, New
York, NY, 10020. 1985. ISBN: 0-671-54634- 1.

(3). Pritikin Longevity Center. 5875 Collins Avenue, Miami Beach,
FL, 33141. (1-800) 327 4914.

(4). Pritikin Longevity Center. 1910 Ocean Front Walk,
Santa Monica, CA, 90405. (1-800) 421 9911.

(5). Ornish, D. **Dr. Dean Ornish's Program for Reversing Heart
Disease**. Ballantine Books, New York, NY. 1990. ISBN: 0-345-37353-7.

(6). The Preventive Medicine Research Institute. 1001 Bridgeway,
Box 305, Sausalito, CA, 94965. (1-800) 328 3738.

(7). Physicians Committee for Responsible Medicine. PO Box 6322,
Washington, DC, 20015. (202) 686 2210. Fax (202) 686 2216.

(8). Bernard, N. D. **The Power of Your Plate**. Book Publishing Co.
PO Box 99, Summertown, TN, 38483. 1990. ISBN 0-913990-69-8.

(9). **The Vegetarian Starter Kit**. Available from: Physicians Committee for Responsible Medicine. PO Box 6322, Washington, DC, 20015. (202) 686 2210.

(10). Klapper, M. **Vegan Nutrition: Pure and Simple**. Gentle World, Inc. PO Box U, Pala, Maui, HI, 96779. 1992. ISBN: 0-9614248-7-7.

(11). McDougall, J. A., and M. A. McDougall. **The McDougall Plan**. New Win Publishing, Inc. PO Box 5159, Dlinton, NJ, 08809. 1983.

(12). American Natural Hygiene Society, Inc. 11816 Race Track Road, Tampa, FL, 33626. (813) 855 6607.

(13). Diamond, H. and M. Diamond. **Fit For Life**. Warner Books, Inc. 1271 Avenue of the Americas, New York, NY, 10020. 1985. ISBN: 0-446-30015-2.

(14). The Hippocrates Health Institute. 1443 Palmdale Court, West Palm Beach, FL, 33411. (1-800) 842 2125.

15. Plastaket Manufacturing Co. 6220 East Highway 12, Lodi, CA, 95240.

(16). Seeds of Change. PO Box 15700, Santa Fe, NM, 87506-5700. (505) 438 8080.

(17). Cell Tech. 1300 Main Street, Klamath Falls, OR, 97601-5914. (503) 882 5406.

(18) Light Force. PO Box 8526, Santa Cruz, CA, 95061. (1-800) 999 5709.

(19). Cole, C. L. **Not Milk . . . Nutmilks**. Woodbridge Press Publishing Co. PO Box 6189, Santa Barbara, CA, 93106. 1990. ISBN: 0-88007-184-2.

(20). SunRider International. 1625 Abalone Ave, Torrance, CA, 90505. (310) 781 8096.

(21). Arrowhead Mills, Inc. PO Box 2059, Hereford, TX, 79045. (1-800) 749 0730.

(22). Omega Nutrition Canada, Inc. 8564 Fraser Street, Vancouver, BC, V5X3Y3. (1-800) 661 3529.

(23). Jaffe Brothers, Inc. PO Box 636. Valley Center, CA, 92082-0636. (619) 749 1133.

(24). Ornish, D. **Eat More, Weigh Less: Dr. Dean Ornish's Life Choice Program for Losing Weight Safely While Eating Abundantly.** Harper Collins Pub., Inc. 10 E. 53rd Street, New York, NY, 10022. 1993. ISBN: 0-06-092545-0.

(25). Diamond, M. **The American Vegetarian Cookbook: From the Fit for Life Kitchen.** Warner Books, Inc. 666 Fifth Avenue, New York, NY, 10103. 1990. ISBN: 0-446-51561-2.

(26). Romano, R. **Dining, in the Raw, Cooking with the Buff**. Nuova Castellosnc, Florence, Italy. 1993. LCCC No 92-96991. For copies send requests to: Rita Romano. 6064 Okeechobee Boulevard, PO Box 170689, West Palm Beach, FL, 33417. (407) 687-3333.

(27). Levine, S. and B. Star. **Living with Live Foods: A Primer**. Star Publishing House. West Palm Beach, FL. 1994. ISBN: 1-884886-02-7. (1-800) 978 2777.

References

(1). Kuczmarski, R. J., et al. *Increasing Prevalence of Overweight Among US Adults: The National Health and Nutrition Examination Survey. 1960-1991*. JAMA. 1994; 272:205-211.

(2). Willett, W. C. *Diet and Health: What Should We Eat?* Science. 1994; 264:532-537.

(3). National Research Council. **Diet and Health Implications for Reducing Chronic Disease Risk**. National Academy Press, Washington, DC. 1989.

(4). Ascherio, A., et al. *A Prospective Study of Nutritional Factors and Hypertension Among US Men*. Circulation. 1992; 86:1475-1484.

(5). Miller, A. B. *Diet in the Etiology of Cancer: A Review*. Eurp J Cancer. 1994; 30A:207-228.

(6). Steinmetz, K. A., et al. *Vegetables, Fruit, and Colon Cancer in the Iowa Women's Health Study.* Am J Epidemiol. 1994;139:1-15.

(7). Bostick, R. M., et al. *Sugar, Meat, and Fat Intake, and Non-Dietary Risk Factors for Colon Cancer Incidence in Iowa Women. (United States).* Cancer Causes Control. 1994; 51:38-52.

(8). Toniolo, P., et al. *Consumption of Meat, Animal Products, Protein and Fat and Risk of Breast Cancer: A Prospective Cohort Study in New York.* Epidemiology. 1994; 5:391-396.

(9). Marchand, L. L. *Animal Fat Consumption and Prostate Cancer: A Prospective Study in Hawaii.* Epidemiology. 1994; 5:276-282.

(10). Block, G., et al. *Fruit, Vegetables, and Cancer Prevention: A Review of the Epidemiological Evidence.* Nutr. Cancer. 1992; 18:1-29.

(11). Willett, W. C. *Vitamin A and Lung Cancer.* Nutr Rev. 1990; 48:201-211.

(12). Darling, L. G. and N. W. Ramsey. *Clinical Review of Dietary Therapy for Rheumatoid Arthritis.* Brit J Rheum. 1993; 32:507-514.

(13). Hankinson, S. E., et al. *Nutrient Intake and Cataract Extraction in Women: Prospective Study.* Brit Med J. 1992; 305:335-339.

(14). Kendall, A., et al. *Weight Loss on a Low-Fat Diet: Consequence of the Imprecision of the Control of Food Intake In Humans.* Am J Clin Nutr. 1991; 53:1124-1129.

(15). Miller, W. *Diet Composition, Energy Intake and Exercise in Relation to Body Fat in Men and Women.* Am J Clin Nutr. 1990; 52:426-430.

(16). Simopoulos, A. P. and T. B. Van Itallie. *Body Weight, Health, and Longevity.* Ann Intern Med. 1984; 100:285-295.

(17). Manson, J. E., et al. *Body Weight and Longevity. A Reassessment.* JAMA. 1987; 257:353-358.

(18). Lee, I-Min, et al. *Body Weight and Mortality: A 27-Year Follow-up of Middle-Aged Men.* JAMA. 1993; 270:2823-2828.

(19). Simpson, H. A *High-Carbohydrate-Leguminous-Fibre Diet Improves All Aspects of Diabetic Control.* Lancet. 1981; 1:1-5.

(20). Anderson, J. W., et al. *Weight Loss and 2-y Follow-up for 80 Morbidly Obese Patients Treated with Intensive Very-Low-Calorie Diet and an Education Program.* Am J Clin Nutr. 1992; 56:244S-246S.

(21). Kramer, F. M., et al. *Long-Term Follow-Up of Behavioral Treatment for Obesity: Patterns of Weight Regain Among Men and Women.* Int J Obesity. 1989; 13:123-136.

(22). Wadden, T. A., et al. *Long-term Effects of Dieting on Resting Metabolic Rate in Obese Outpatients.* JAMA. 1990; 264:707-711.

(23). Howe, G. A. *A Cohort Study of Fat Intake and Risk of Breast Cancer.* J Nutr Clin Res. 1991; 83:336-340.

(24). Willet, W. *Dietary Fat and the Risk of Breast Cancer*. N Engl J Med. 1987; 316:22-28.

(25). Keusch, G. T., et al. *Ecology of the Gastrointestinal Tract*. p 1645. In: Berk, E. J., ed. **Gastroenterology**. W. B. Saunders, Co. Philadelphia, PA. 1985, Vol 3, 4th ed.

(26). Gerstein, H. C. *Cow's Milk Exposure and Type I Diabetes Mellitus*. Diabetes Care. 1994; 17:13-19.

(27). Ursin, G., et al. *Milk Consumption and Cancer Incidence: A Norwegian Prospective Study*. Brit J Cancer. 1990; 61:454-459.

(28). Cramer, D. W. *Lactase Persistence and Milk Consumption as Determinants of Ovarian Cancer Risk*. Am J Epidemiol. 1989; 130:904-910.

(29). Leonard, R. E. *Home and Abroad, FDA Befriends Chemical Firms*. Nutr Week. 1994; 4:4-5.

(30). Guyton, A. C. **Textbook of Medical Physiology**. W. B. Saunders Co., Philadelphia, PA. 1991, 8th ed. p. 769.

(31). Chaney, S.G. *Principles of Nutrition I: Macronutrients*. p 1095-1098. In: Devlin, T. M., ed. **Textbook of Biochemistry. With Clinical Correlations**. Wiley-Liss, New York, NY. 1992, 3rd ed.

(32). Ibid. p 1098.

(33). Ibid. p 1098.

(34). Gaziano, J. M. *Antioxidant Vitamins and Coronary Artery Disease Risk.* Am J Med. 1994; 97(suppl 3A): 3A-18S-3A-21S.

(35). Hennekens, C. H. *Antioxidant Vitamins and Cancer.* Am J Med. 1994; 97(suppl 3A):3A-2S-3A-4S.

(36). Steinmetz, K. A. and J. D. Potter. *Vegetables, Fruit and Cancer. I. Epidemiology.* Cancer Causes Control. 1991; 2:325-357.

(37). Greenberg, E. R. *A Clinical Trial of Antioxidant Vitamins to Prevent Colorectal Adenoma.* N Engl J Med. 1994; 331:141-147.

(38). Ibid. p 146.

(39). Schardt, D. *Phytochemicals: Plants Against Cancer.* Nutrition Action Health Letter. 1994; 21:7-13.

(40). Geleijuse, J. M., et. al. *Reduction in Blood Pressure with a Low Sodium, High Potassium, High Magnesium Salt in Older Subjects with Mild to Moderate Hypertension.* Brit. Med. J. 1994; 309:436-440.

Chapter 4

Resources

(1). Nightingale Conant. 7300 North Lehigh Avenue, Niles, IL, 60714. (1-800) 525 9000.

(2). Avatar. The Star's Edge Consultant. 900 Markham Woods Road, Longwood, FL, 32779. (407) 788 3090.

(3). Insight Seminars. 2101 Wilshire Boulevard, Santa Monica, CA, 90403. (310) 829-919.

(4) Lifespring Corporate Office. 161 Mitchell Boulevard, San Rafael, CA, 94903. (415) 479 7873.

(5). Global Relationship Centers, Inc. 16101 Stewart Rd, Austin, TX, 78734. (1-800) 333 3896.

(6). Esalen Institute. Big Sur, CA, 93920-9616. (408) 667 3000.

(7). Omega Institute. 260 Lake Drive, Rhinebeck, NY, 12572-3212. (914) 266 4301.

(8). Kripalu Center. Box 793, Lenox, MA, 01240. (413) 448 3400.

(9). Self Talk Cassettes. 4355 East University, Suite 107-18, Mesa, AZ, 85205. (1-800) 255 1732.

(10). Sound R_X. 524 San Anselmo Avenue, Suite 700, San Anselmo, CA, 94960. (1-800) 876 8637.

(11). The Monroe Institute. Route 1, Box 175, Faber, VA, 22938-9749. (804) 361 1500.

References

(1). Peck, M. S. **The Road Less Traveled. A New Psychology of Love, Traditional Values and Spiritual Growth**. Simon and Schuster. New York, NY. 1978. ISBN: 0-671-24086-2.

(2). Campbell, J. **The Power of Myth. With Bill Moyers**. Doubleday. New York, NY. 1988. ISBN: 0-385-24773-7.

(3). Fromm, E. **The Art of Loving**. Harper & Brothers Pub., New York, NY. 1956.

Index*

INDEX 🌐

INDEX 🌐

*(f)=Figure, (t)=Table

Dear Reader,

Dr. Young and the Tri Health staff would greatly appreciate your feedback on this book. . . both good and bad . . . by filling out and returning this form. Your comments will help Tri Health improve new editions of this book and create new products to fulfill our mission: to provide resources for people to help themselves achieve Total Well Being. Thank you very much!

Overall:	Very Poor	Poor	Average	Good	Very Good
Artistic Presence	❑	❑	❑	❑	❑
User Friendliness	❑	❑	❑	❑	❑
Content	❑	❑	❑	❑	❑
Credibility	❑	❑	❑	❑	❑

Book Content:					
General Health Care	❑	❑	❑	❑	❑
Exercise	❑	❑	❑	❑	❑
Nutrition	❑	❑	❑	❑	❑
Stress Management	❑	❑	❑	❑	❑

Additional Interest In:	Yes	No
Exercise Manual	❑	❑
Recipes	❑	❑
Audiotapes	❑	❑
Videotapes	❑	❑

Comments: _____
_____
_____
_____

Name:_____

Address:_____

City:_____ State:_____ Zip_____

Day Phone:_____ Night Phone:_____

For information on lectures, seminars workshops or to order additional copies of this book call: 1-800 DR YOUNG (379 6864).